Tucholsky Wagner Zola Scott Sydow Freud Schlegel
Turgenev Wallace Fonatne
Twain Walther von der Vogelweide Fouqué Friedrich II. von Preußen
Weber Freiligrath Frey
Fechner Fichte Weiße Rose von Fallersleben Kant Ernst Frommel
Hölderlin Richthofen
Engels Fielding Eichendorff Tacitus Dumas
Fehrs Faber Flaubert Eliasberg Ebner Eschenbach
Feuerbach Maximilian I. von Habsburg Fock Eliot Zweig
Ewald Vergil
Goethe Elisabeth von Österreich London
Mendelssohn Balzac Shakespeare Dostojewski Ganghofer
Trackl Lichtenberg Rathenau Doyle Gjellerup
Mommsen Stevenson Hambruch
Thoma Tolstoi Lenz Hanrieder Droste-Hülshoff
Dach Verne von Arnim Hägele Hauff Humboldt
Karrillon Reuter Rousseau Hagen Hauptmann Gautier
Garschin
Damaschke Defoe Hebbel Baudelaire
Descartes Hegel Kussmaul Herder
Wolfram von Eschenbach Darwin Dickens Schopenhauer Rilke George
Bronner Melville Grimm Jerome Bebel Proust
Campe Horváth Aristoteles Federer
Bismarck Vigny Barlach Voltaire Herodot
Gengenbach Heine
Storm Casanova Tersteegen Gilm Grillparzer Georgy
Chamberlain Lessing Langbein Gryphius
Brentano Lafontaine
Strachwitz Claudius Schiller Kralik Iffland Sokrates
Bellamy Schilling
Katharina II. von Rußland Gerstäcker Raabe Gibbon Tschechow
Löns Hesse Hoffmann Gogol Wilde Gleim Vulpius
Luther Heym Hofmannsthal Klee Hölty Morgenstern Goedicke
Roth Heyse Klopstock Kleist
Luxemburg Puschkin Homer Mörike Musil
La Roche Horaz
Machiavelli Kierkegaard Kraft Kraus
Navarra Aurel Musset Moltke
Nestroy Marie de France Lamprecht Kind Kirchhoff Hugo
Nietzsche Nansen Laotse Ipsen Liebknecht
Marx Lassalle Gorki Klett Leibniz Ringelnatz
von Ossietzky May vom Stein Lawrence Irving
Petalozzi Knigge
Platon Pückler Michelangelo Kafka
Sachs Poe Liebermann Kock
de Sade Praetorius Mistral Zetkin Korolenko

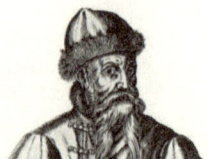

The publishing house tradition has created the series **TREDITION CLASSICS**. It contains classical literature works from over two thousand years. Most of these titles have been out of print and off the bookstore shelves for decades.

The book series is intended to preserve the cultural legacy and to promote the timeless works of classical literature. As a reader of a **TREDITION CLASSICS** book, the reader supports the mission to save many of the amazing works of world literature from oblivion.

The symbol of **TREDITION CLASSICS** is Johannes Gutenberg (1400 – 1468), the inventor of movable type printing.

With the series, tradition intends to make thousands of international literature classics available in printed format again – worldwide.

All books are available at book retailers worldwide in paperback and in hardcover. For more information please visit: www.tredition.com

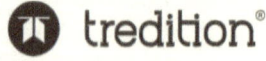

tradition was established in 2006 by Sandra Latusseck and Soenke Schulz. Based in Hamburg, Germany, tradition offers publishing solutions to authors and publishing houses, combined with worldwide distribution of printed and digital book content. tradition is uniquely positioned to enable authors and publishing houses to create books on their own terms and without conventional manufacturing risks.

For more information please visit: www.tredition.com

The Four Epochs of Woman's Life
a study in hygiene

Anna M. (Anna Mary) Galbraith

Imprint

This book is part of the TREDITION CLASSICS series.

Author: Anna M. (Anna Mary) Galbraith
Cover design: toepferschumann, Berlin (Germany)

Publisher: tredition GmbH, Hamburg (Germany)
ISBN: 978-3-8491-8802-3

www.tredition.com
www.tredition.de

Copyright:
The content of this book is sourced from the public domain.

The intention of the TREDITION CLASSICS series is to make world literature in the public domain available in printed format. Literary enthusiasts and organizations worldwide have scanned and digitally edited the original texts. tredition has subsequently formatted and redesigned the content into a modern reading layout. Therefore, we cannot guarantee the exact reproduction of the original format of a particular historic edition. Please also note that no modifications have been made to the spelling, therefore it may differ from the orthography used today.

"As in a building
Stone rests on stone, and wanting the foundation
All would be wanting, so in human life
Each action rests on the foregoing event
That made it possible, but is forgotten
And buried in the earth."

— LONGFELLOW.

INTRODUCTORY NOTE

IT has been well said that the bulwarks of a nation are the mothers. Any contribution to the physical, and hence the mental, perfection of woman should be welcomed alike by her own sex, by the thoughtful citizen, by the political economist, and by the hygienist. Observation of the truths, expressed in a modest, pleasing, and conclusive manner, in the essay of Dr. Galbraith contribute to this end. These truths should be known by every woman, and I gladly commend the essay to their thoughtful consideration.

JOHN H. MUSSER, M.D.,

*Late Professor of Clinical Medicine
in the University of Pennsylvania.*

PREFACE TO THE SECOND EDITION.

THE author takes this opportunity to thank the medical profession and the laity for the very cordial reception which has been tendered the first edition of this small volume.

The necessity for the use of technical expressions in a book written expressly for the laity must always be a matter of regret. And only those who have attempted to write a similar work can fully appreciate the truth of Herbert Spencer's remark, that "Nothing is so difficult as to write an elementary book on scientific subjects."

The author has added to this edition a section on "The Hygiene of Puberty," one on "Hemorrhage at the Menopause a Significant Symptom of Cancer," and one on "The Hygiene of the Menopause."

ANNA M. GALBRAITH.

15 WEST NINETY-FIRST STREET, NEW YORK.

PREFACE.

> "Ignorance is the curse of God;
> Knowledge, the wings wherewith we fly to heaven."
>
> — *"Henry VI."*

PERFECT health is essential to perfect happiness. The greater the knowledge of the laws of nature, and the more closely these laws are lived up to, so much nearer "ideal" will be the health and happiness of the individual. Hence the necessity that these same laws should be as familiar to the adult man and woman as the alphabet. Further, with our present knowledge of the certain suffering, disease, and death that are bred by ignorance of all these subjects, it is little less than criminal to allow girls to reach the age of puberty without the slightest knowledge of the menstrual function; young women to be married in total ignorance of the ethics of married life; women to become mothers without any conception of the duties of motherhood; other women, as the time approaches, to live in dread apprehension of "the change of life;" and many women unnecessarily to succumb to disease at this time.

The masses of women have at last awakened to a sense of the awful penalties which they have paid for their ignorance of all those laws of nature which govern their physical being, and to feel keenly the necessity for instruction at least in the fundamental principles which underlie the various epochs of their lives; and it is in response to a widespread demand that this small volume has been written.

This is preeminently the day of preventive medicine; and the physician who can prevent the origin of disease is a greater benefactor than the one who can lessen the mortality or suffering after the disease has occurred.

ANNA M. GALBRAITH.

15 WEST NINETY-FIRST STREET, NEW YORK.

CONTENTS

INTRODUCTION

EDUCATION AS THE CONTROLLING FACTOR IN THE PHYSICAL LIFE OF WOMAN

Huxley's Definition of Education; the Correlation of Mind and Body; the Emotional Nature; Age for Going to School; the Effect of the Study of the Scientific Branches; Industrial Education

PART I. — MAIDENHOOD

CHAPTER I.

PUBERTY

Sexual Development; Age of Puberty; Physical Changes at Puberty; First Onset of Menstruation; Psychic Changes at Puberty

CHAPTER II.

HYGIENE OF PUBERTY

Home Life; Corsets; Shoes; Underwear; Nutrition; Diet; Water; Constipation; School Life; Spinal Curvature; Exercise; Walking; Running

CHAPTER III.

ANATOMY OF THE FEMALE GENERATIVE ORGANS

The Vulva; the Hymen; Condition of the Hymen as a Proof of Virginity; the Bladder; Vagina; Uterus; Respiratory Movements of the Uterus; Fallopian Tubes; Ovaries

CHAPTER IV.

PHYSIOLOGY OF THE FEMALE GENERATIVE ORGANS

Ovulation; Etiology of Menstruation; Uterine Nerve-supply; the Function of the Uterus; Stages of the Menstrual Cycle; Average Duration of the Menstrual Flow; Character of the Flow; Relation of Ovulation to Menstruation; the Menstrual Wave; Definition of Menstruation; Premonitory Symptoms of the Flow; Hygiene of Menstruation

CHAPTER V.

THE ANOMALIES OF MENSTRUATION

Menorrhagia and Metrorrhagia; Dysmenorrhea; Amenorrhea; Leucorrhea; Pruritus Vulva

CHAPTER VI.

THE MARRIAGE QUESTION

Herbert Spencer's Definition of Love; What Constitutes a Suitable Husband; Best Age for Marriage; Shall Cousins Marry? Contraindications to Marriage; Do Reformed Profligates Make Good Husbands? the Proper Length of Time for the Engagement; the Right Time of the Year to Marry; the Selection of the Wedding Day

PART II. — MARRIAGE

CHAPTER VII.

THE ETHICS OF MARRIED LIFE

The Wedding Journey; the Ethics of Married Life; Shall Husband and Wife Occupy the Same Bed? the Consummation of Marriage; the Marital Relation; Times when Marital Relations Should be Suspended

CHAPTER VIII.

SEXUAL INSTINCT IN WOMEN

Sexual Instinct in Women; Excessive Coitus; Causes of Sexual Excitability

CHAPTER IX.

STERILITY

Sterility; the Prevention of Conception and the Limitation of Offspring; the Crime of Abortion; Infidelity in Women

PART III.— MATERNITY

CHAPTER X.

PREGNANCY

Nature of Conception; Pregnancy Defined; Duration of Pregnancy; the Signs of Pregnancy; Quickening; the Determination of Sex at Will; the Influence of the Male Sexual Element on the Fernale Organism; Heredity; Hygiene of Pregnancy; Causes of Miscarriage

CHAPTER XI.

THE CONFINMENT

Preparation for the Confinement; Signs of Approaching Labor; Symptoms of Actual Labor; The Confinement-bed; the Process of Labor

CHAPTER XII.

THE LYING-IN

Management of the Lying-in; Lactation; Nursing

CHAPTER XIII.

THE NEW-BORN INFANT

The Infant's Toilet; the Crib; Feeding of Infants; the Wet-nurse; Artificial Feeding; Characteristics of Healthy Infants; the Stools; Constipation; Urination; Teething

PART IV.— THE MENOPAUSE

CHAPTER XIV.

THE MENOPAUSE

Average Duration of the Menstrual Function; Duration of Menopause; the Menopause; General Phenomena of the Menopause; Prominent Symptoms of Menopause; Pathologic Conditions of Menopause; Hemorrhage at the Menopause a Significant Symptom of Cancer; Causes of Suffering at Menopause

CHAPTER XV.

HYGIENE OF THE MENOPAUSE

Diet; Constipation; Stimulants; the Kidneys; Skin; Turkish Baths; Massage; Exercise; Profuse Menstruation; Hemorrhage; Mental Therapeutics

CHAPTER XVI.

HINTS FOR HOME TREATMENT

Indigestion; Constipation; Enemas; Diarrhea; Vaginal Douché, Baths; Headache; Fainting; Hemorrhage

GLOSSARY

INTRODUCTION.

EDUCATION AS THE CONTROLLING FACTOR IN THE PHYSICAL LIFE OF WOMAN.

Huxley's Definition of Education; the Correlation of Mind and Body; the Emotional Nature; Age for Going to School; the Effect of the Study of tuse Scientific Branches; Industrial Education.

> "What is man,
> If his chief good, and market of his time,
> Be but to sleep and feed? A beast; no more.
> Sure, He that made us with such large discourse,
> Looking before and after, gave us not
> That capability and godlike reason
> To fust in us unused."
>
> — *"Hamlet."*

THE word education is here used in its broadest sense, and is meant to include the physical, mental, intellectual, and industrial. Huxley's definition is as follows: "Education is the instruction of the intellect in the laws of nature, under which I include not only things and their forces, but men and their ways; and the fashioning of their affections and of the will into an earnest and living desire to move in harmony with these laws. That man, I think, has had a liberal education who has been so trained in his youth that his body is the ready servant of his will, and does with ease and pleasure all the work that, as a mechanism, it is capable of; whose intellect is a clear, cold, logic engine, to be turned to any kind of work, to spin the gossamers as well as to forge the anchors of the mind; whose mind is stored with the great and fundamental truths of nature and the laws of her operations; one whose passions are trained to come to heel by a vigorous will, the servant of a tender conscience; one who has learned to love all beauty, whether of nature or of art, to hate all vileness, and to respect others as himself."

The Correlation of Mind and Body. — It is of the utmost importance that the mutual reaction of mind and body upon each other should be thoroughly understood. This reaction is so constant, so intricate, and so complex that it is at times difficult to say which is cause and which effect. Does the depressed state of the mind cause the indigestion, or is a torpid liver the real seat of the melancholia?

The brain is the most delicately constructed organ in the entire body. In the lower animals the brain is simply the great nerve-center which, with its prolongation the spinal cord, presides over all the functions of life which differentiate the animal from the vegetable. In the human being the brain is much more highly developed and complicated; and is, in addition, the seat of the mind, the intellect, and the affections. Like all the other tissues of the body, the brain receives its nourishment from the blood-vessels which pass through it, and its healthy maintenance is in a direct ratio to the condition of its blood-supply.

A most interesting psychologic study is found in the case of cerebral paralysis of young children, where there is mental defect amounting to stupidity or imbecility, accompanied by extensive paralysis of the body, so that the child is not able to sit up. With the gradual improvement of the physical condition, so that the muscles become firm and the child can sit, stand, and even walk, there is a corresponding mental development; from being stupid and dull, the expression of the face brightens and becomes intelligent; the child talks quite as well as other children of its age, and sometimes becomes really intellectually precocious. Here we see the development of the brain as a direct result of the improved physical condition. In certain cases of insanity, on the contrary, we find that the wasting away of the body results from the disease of the brain, *i. e.*, the disease of the brain has wrought the wreck of the body.

From these pathologic studies, or studies of how the diseased state of the brain and body may be overcome by physical development, on the one hand, and, on the other hand, how the healthy body may be wrecked by disease of the brain, we will turn to a consideration of the effect of the development of the mind and intellect upon the physical health.

On a girl's entering Vassar College an exact and detailed physical examination is made by the resident physician, a health record is kept during her stay there, and at the time of her graduation a final physical examination is made. As a result of these statistics Dr.

Thelberg says: "These statistics, now covering a number of years, show that not only can girls profitably take a college education, that is accomplished; but will prove that grave physical imperfections can be corrected in the period between eighteen and twenty-two years of age, coincidently with the development of the mind along the lines of college work; the college work, if not excessive in amount, being a real and most important factor in the physical development."

But a still more striking proof can be cited of the beneficial result of mental and intellectual occupation upon the bodily health. At Vassar a great deal of attention is very properly paid to general hygiene and the physical development, in addition to the natural advantages of outdoor life in the country.

Take, for example, a woman's medical college located in the city: the four years' course places the greatest strain on both mind and body; practically no time is left for recreation, and very much too little time is spent in sleep; the amount of exercise taken is the minimum. Yet in spite of all these disadvantages under which the young women labor, a great many of them who enter far below par in health, or, indeed, on the fair road to become chronic invalids, graduate very greatly improved in health.

The Emotional Nature.— Formerly much more than now, owing to the defective methods of her education and mode of life, the emotional nature of woman was allowed to run riot. The child was coddled; the girl was allowed to grow up without any of the discipline which young men receive in their college and business life, and little or no attention was paid to her physical development. The woman naturally became a bundle of nerves, highly irritable, unreasonable, and hysterical. All this reacted in the most detrimental manner upon her physical health.

The seed for much of this emotional hyperesthesia is sown in childhood. From birth until the end of the eighth year should be one grand holiday. During this time the child develops very rapidly, especially during the first two years of life. And at the end of the eighth year the brain has attained to within a few ounces of its full weight. The muscular system has been developed together with the coordination of motion. The child has learned to use a language fairly well; she has developed an excellent memory and is most inquisitive and acquisitive.

Another method for undermining the healthy tone of the nervous system is the intricate dances taught very young children and then placing them on public exhibition, where they are wrought up to the highest pitch. From a purely medical standpoint, children under eight years of age should not be allowed to take dancing lessons. After this age a moderate amount of dancing in a well-ventilated room is good exercise.

Children's parties belong in the same category, and, on account of the injurious effects on the nervous system, should be tabooed. They are too exciting, and cause an overstimulation of the nervous system and a precocious childhood and puberty.

Instead of rearing an oversensitive hot - house plant that must be fragile in the extreme, strive to rear a sturdy plant that can hold its own amid the storms. The child should spend as much of its life as possible in the open air, and in the warm months live out-of-doors. City children should be taken to the seashore or country to spend several months every summer. Together with outdoor sports, gymnastics adapted to the age of the child should be begun early and continued throughout life. Good muscular development is attended with good digestion and a well-balanced nervous system.

Until after the twelfth year there should be absolutely no difference between the physical, mental, or industrial education of girls and boys. And, still further, they should be encouraged to have their sports together; this will improve the girls physically and broaden them mentally, and will do a great deal to take the rough edges off the boys. After this age it will be wise to allow slight barriers to grow up, without calling the attention of any one to the fact, that will cause the companionship to be less free and unrestrained.

Age for Going to School.— Although the child may be allowed to go to kindergarten long before this time, it should not be allowed to enter the school-room before eight years of age. And from eight to twelve years, not more than four hours a day should be spent in study. After this time it may be put down more closely to intellectual work; but no more mental work should be required than will enable the girl to enter college at eighteen. And eighteen years of age is as young as any girl should be allowed to go to college; after this age the mind is more matured and acquires knowledge more easily than before, while the development of the body is less rapid. The physical system has become more stable. The literature indulged in by girls under eighteen years of age should be most carefully selected.

The Effect of the Study of the Scientific Branches.— A knowledge of the laws of nature is essential to health; hence the necessity for the study of the natural sciences— anatomy, physiology, chemistry, physics, and zoology. Aside from the intrinsic value of this knowledge, it is almost universally conceded that these studies develop the judgment; and no one will have the temerity to deny that a lack of judgment must undermine the health as well as the success and happiness of the individual.

Industrial Education.— When it is considered how intimate are the relations between the physical and the psychic states, and how often the psychic condition leads to actual disease, and that often of the most incurable type, it needs no demonstration that a mental occupation which will take the woman out of herself is a physical necessity. Therefore when the girl has reached the subjective limit of her intellectual education,— that is, when she has reached the limit of her capacity or taste,— it is essential to her physical well-being that she should turn her attention to some industrial occupation. This may be housekeeping or any other occupation for which she has taste or talent. A healthy mental occupation is an absolute necessity to prevent the individual from becoming self-centered. And to become self-centered is the first step on the certain road to chronic invalidism.

A most important part of an education is the knowledge of how to procure the most perfect development of the body possible, and how to maintain the health. This has not been touched upon here, since the outlines for the general physical education have already been given in "Hygiene and Physical Culture for Women,"* and the present volume concerns itself only with the four critical epochs of woman's life.

* By Anna M. Galbraith, M. D.; published by Dodd, Mead & Co.

With this broad view of an education, as a means to procure the best physique possible; a mind disciplined to meet to the greatest advantage all the vicissitudes of life; an intellect developed along the lines of its greatest possibilities; and an occupation chosen in accordance with the tastes and talents of the individual; it becomes an incontrovertible fact that *the education is the controlling factor* in the physical life of every woman.

> "Be not simply good; be good for something."
>
> THOREAU.

PART I.— MAIDENHOOD.

CHAPTER I.

PUBERTY.

Sexual Development; Age of Puberty; Physical Changes at Puberty; First Onset of Menstruation; Psychic Changes at Puberty.

> "Self-reverence, self-knowledge, self-control,
> These three alone lead life to sovereign power."
>
> — "ŒEnone."

Sexual Development.— Sexual development goes on during all the years of childhood, but is not complete in the female sex until between the twenty-second and the twenty-fifth year. If the child has no inherited taint, and has been properly educated morally, physically, and intellectually, it must follow that the structural development of the pelvic organs has been normal; and normal organs always perform their functions perfectly.

The commencement of the ovarian function does not cause any more profound change in the system and habits than does dentition. The various epochs of life are generally spoken of as if they were paroxysmal— as though they were separated by some tremendous chasm, which had to be leapt over or fallen into. Nature makes no such egregious blunders; preparations for every change in life have been going on for a very long time before the evidences of such change become manifest.

In a healthy girl the psychic and physical changes incident to puberty occur so gradually as to escape the girl's own notice. The first and, if the girl has not been properly prepared for it, always startling change is the appearance of the menstrual flow. The mother who has not told her daughter of this coming change in her life before it is due has committed a serious error; it is no uncommon occurrence for girls who know nothing of this function to get into a tub of cold water to stop the flow; and if they stay in long enough, it generally does stop, and the girl's health may be ruined for life.

The opinion of Dr. Ely van de Warker is that "if healthy ovulation is the outcome of healthy childhood, the function will obey the law of periodicity year by year, and all this time the young woman will be able to sustain uninterrupted physical and intellectual work as well as the young man. Not that the laws of health may be violated with impunity at puberty or any other time of a woman's life; but a law of health is no more binding upon a young woman than it is upon a young man; and there really is no such thing as one law for women and another for men."

Age of Puberty.— In the temperate regions the age of puberty is reached between the ages of twelve and fourteen years. The girl is then said to be nubile; that is, as soon as menstruation appears it is possible for her to bear children; but she is by no means sufficiently developed to do so, as she herself will not be completely developed physically or mentally before the age of twenty-two or twenty-five years.

Physical Changes at Puberty.— The physical changes that gradually take place, beginning at the time of puberty, are: the breasts, pelvis, and neck enlarge; hair develops over the pubis and in the arm-pits; the voice alters. As a rule, women continue to grow in stature until the twenty-fifth year. It is said that brunettes develop sooner than blondes, and that large women develop more slowly than women of small stature; city girls develop younger than girls brought up in the country. Whatever stimulates the emotions causes a premature development of the sexual organs; as children's parties, late hours, sensational novels, loose stories, the drama and the ballroom, talk of beaux, of love and marriage, and children being surrounded with the atmosphere of riper years. It is generally believed that early stimulation of the sexual instincts leads to the premature establishment of puberty, as do also spiced foods and alcoholic beverages.

First Onset of Menstruation.— Sometimes the first menstrual discharge appears suddenly, lasts for a few days, and then stops; it may appear after an interval of two or three weeks, or not for several months. If for several months the flow appears at the regular time, and the quantity is about the same as the first, the menstrual habit may be said to be established. The mode of onset varies considerably within the limits of health. So long as the general health remains good, no anxiety need be felt in regard to the establishment of the menstrual function.

In other cases there may be a discharge of blood at the first period, and none afterward for several months; in other words, menstruation may be established suddenly, intermittently, or gradually. It must be remembered that certain pathologic conditions cause many disturbances connected with the onset of puberty.

Psychic Changes at Puberty.— The angular, gawky feeling gradually disappears; the girl becomes self-conscious; new impulses arise, and she gives up many of the hoydenish ways of childhood. The girl's imagination is more lively, and just at this time mathematics form an excellent subject for mental occupation. The girl now begins to question the whys and wherefores, and demands reasons for the course that is laid out for her, and is full of ideas of her own; so that while as a child she had accepted almost unquestioningly the commands of her parents, she can be managed now only through the power of reason. And this is just as it should be, for the girl has reached the years of discretion, and now is the time when her reason and judgment are capable of rapid cultivation.

CHAPTER II.

HYGIENE OF PUBERTY.

Home Life; Corsets; Shoes; Underwear; Nutrition; Diet; Water; Constipation; School Life; Spinal Curvature; Exercise; Walking; Running.

"Every man is the architect of his own fortune."

PSEUDO-SALLUST.

Home Life.— With beginning menstruation the equilibrium of the body is very easily disturbed, so that even in the case of the healthy girl some precautions should be taken and a rational regime should be adhered to; while in the case of the delicate girl a still more careful attention will have to be directed toward her weak points, in order that she may develop into a healthy woman.

For every girl at this time of life home is preeminently the place; so that she may not only have the benefit of a mother's watchful care, but also lead a life as free from conventionalities and as much in the open air as possible. No girl should be sent away to school at this period of rapid growth and development; nor should girls of the working classes, when it can possibly be avoided, be sent out to fill positions as clerks in illy ventilated stores, in factories, or as domestics. If a girl can be kept at home until she is eighteen years old, she will be a much stronger, healthier woman than would otherwise be possible.

Corsets.— At this period of life it is particularly necessary that the clothing should be warm and at the same time sufficiently loose to prevent the constriction of any part of the body. And whatever the adult woman may elect to do in the matter of wearing corsets herself, she does her young daughter an irreparable injury by constricting and moulding her growing body in these corset-splints. Corsets placed on the young girl interfere with the functions of circulation, respiration, digestion, and of the pelvic organs, also with muscular development. In addition to all this, the girl is handicapped in taking all outdoor exercises and athletic sports.

The lungs, heart, and great blood-vessels are placed in and completely fill an air-tight, distensiblecage, which is most distensible at its base.

The least chest girth of the adult woman— that is, the under-arm girth around the chest— that is consistent with health is twenty-eight inches; and this girth must be enlarged three inches in forced inspiration. In ordinary respiration the waist expansion should be one-half to one inch, while during great muscular activity it should be from one and a half to three or four inches. One-third of the lungs lie below the point of beginning corset pressure, so that with tight corsets this amount of lung substance must be more or less useless.

It is self-evident that any restriction placed about the waist, by preventing the full expansion of the ribs and the descent of the diaphragm, will further embarrass the heart's action by diminishing the amount of room it has to work in, at the same time that it diminishes the amount of oxygen which is inspired. Fresh air is by far the most important part of the daily food. It is in the lungs that the blood throws off its carbonic acid and other impurities; but it is able to do this only when the lungs are supplied with an abundance of oxygen. Every inch which a woman adds to her chest measure adds to the measure of her days.

Great physical injury has followed women playing lawn-tennis while tightly corseted. And although dancing is a much milder exercise, since it frequently takes place in an overheated and poorly ventilated room, fatal results occasionally occur from the same cause.

Standing erect calls into action almost all the muscles of the trunk, neck, and lower extremities. So long as the line of gravity falls within the area of the feet, the muscular effort required is so slight that it is little more than the tonicity contained in all living muscle. The greater the displacement of the line of gravity, the greater the muscular effort required to maintain the equilibrium of the body. Up to a certain extent, exercising the muscle develops the strength and size of the muscle. On the other hand, when a muscle within the body is unused, it wastes; when used within certain limits, it grows. But when the corset splint is applied to the body of the young girl, it supplants the functions of the abdominal and back muscles, which is to hold the trunk erect, and these muscles gradually grow weak and waste. And so the liability to the various spinal curvatures is increased.

The original object of the corset was to give greater prominence to the hips and abdomen. But fashions change! In "the French figure" or straight-front corset now in vogue the pelvis is tilted forward, producing a sinking in of the abdomen and a marked prominence of the hips and sacrum, necessitating a compensatory curve of the spine which increases the curvature forward at the small of the back— a deformity which, a few years ago, women were going to orthopedic surgeons to have corrected. In this attitude the line passing through the centre of gravity strikes the heels, the knees are hyper-extended, and the muscles of the calves and thighs are rendered tense.

By interfering with the muscular development and digestion, the girl is very apt to become angular, flat-chested, anemic, and to have a muddy complexion. And so the corset really defeats the object for which it was put on— that of giving the girl a good figure and enhancing her beauty.

There is no objection to girls wearing any of the various forms of hygienic waists now on the market.

Shoes.— The feet are the part of the body to come in contact with the greatest degree of cold, whether on the floor of the house or the pavement of the street. Hence it is a matter of prime importance to the entire body that the feet should be properly clad.

The thick-soled, flat-heeled shoes which became popular with bicycling and golf are most hygienic, and it is highly desirable that this style of shoe should be adhered to for outdoor exercise.

Underwear.— In our cold and changeable climate the most suitable undergarment is the "combination" woolen undersuit, which reaches from neck to ankles and has long sleeves. Much greater warmth is afforded when the undersuit is moderately tight fitting. Such a suit should be worn the entire year, the grade of weight being adapted to the season.

Nutrition.— The nutrition of the body is dependent on the food supply, digestion and excretion. The growing girl should eat more than the adult woman, because of her more active life and of the fact that the food which she takes must not only replace the worn-out material of the body, but also provide new material needed for growth. Insufficient food and food of defective quality and composition work proportionately for more harm during the growing age.

The full adult weight is not attained before the twenty-fifth year. When the final growth of the body and development of the vital organs is completed, the function of food is simply to replace waste with new material and to furnish material for the development of force.

Diet.— The diet should be a mixed one, consisting of the various kinds of fresh meats, fish, milk, eggs, poultry, vegetables, fruit, and fat in the shape of cream, butter, and the fat of beef and mutton. Animal food improves the condition of the muscles, which are made firmer than they would be through a vegetable diet. Meat in general has a more stimulating effect upon the system and is more strengthening than vegetable food, and it gives rise to a sensation of energy and activity. The common estimate is that meat should occupy one-fourth and vegetable food three-fourths of a mixed diet.

Common salt in moderate quantity is essential, but all highly spiced or seasoned foods should be avoided, also pickles and vinegar. All "sweets" are harmful, because they destroy the appetite for other things and upset the digestion. Tea and coffee should be tabooed, as well as all alcoholic beverages.

Good digestion depends for the most part on serving the meals at the same hour every day, eating leisurely, and masticating the food well. There is a great tendency on the part of the school girl to sleep late in the morning, then "bolt" her breakfast in order to get to school in time. Nothing could be more pernicious to the digestion, unless it is the eternal nibbling of candy.

A healthy girl needs nothing between meals. A delicate girl will be the better for a glass of milk in the middle of the morning and at bed-time; or pure beef juice may be given instead.

Water.— Water is needed to keep the kidneys properly flushed. The amount of urine secreted during the twenty-four hours should be three pints. Of course it will be less than this if the quantity of water is insufficient. In addition to the urine about ten ounces of water are lost from the surface of the lungs, and eighteen ounces from the skin, making a total of about five pints; and this quantity of water must be taken daily in order to maintain the equilibrium of the body. The solid food of a mixed diet contains from fifty to sixty per cent. of water, so that about twenty-five ounces of water are taken into the system daily as an integral part of the food. In addition, three pints more should be taken as plain water. The bladder acts as a reservoir for the urine, and should be emptied at least three or four times a day.

Constipation.— In order to keep the digestive system in good condition, the refuse matter which collects in the lower bowel must be evacuated *every* day. And in order to secure this regular bowel movement, regularity in the time of going to the toilet is a prime necessity. And now is the time when the habits of a lifetime are being formed. If a tendency to constipation exists, it can almost always be overcome by increasing the amount of fruit and vegetables eaten, also by eating cracked wheat, oatmeal, corn and graham bread; all of which increase the peristaltic action of the intestines. The small amount of water taken by girls and women is another fertile source of constipation.

School Life.— When it is considered that fully one-half of the girl's waking hours are spent in school or in study preparing for school, it becomes evident that the girl's attitude at her desk should be the correct one. The malpositions at the desk are the most frequent cause of lateral curvatures, round shoulders, and flat chests. And these deformities are more common in girls than they are in boys.

The common faults of the desk and seat leading to these malpositions are unsuitable shape of the back of the seat, too great a distance between the seat and the desk, and the incorrect slope of the desk.

The edge of the desk should slightly project over the edge of the chair. The top of the desk should incline downward about ten degrees toward the student, and be low enough to allow the forearm to rest on it without raising the shoulder. The seat should be sufficiently deep to support almost the entire thigh, and close enough to the floor to allow the soles of the feet to rest firmly on it. The back of the chair should be arched so as to support the hollow of the back, and should reach just above the lower part of the shoulder-blades, and so make it easy and comfortable for even a weakly child to sit upright.

If the seat is too high, the feet do not rest on the floor, and so the girl does not get the proper aid from the legs and feet to maintain an erect position. If the desk is too high, the elbow can rest on it only by curving the spine and raising the shoulder. The work is brought too close to the eyes and causes extra strain. If the desk is too low, the child stoops over it and becomes round-shouldered, and there is a tendency to become short-sighted.

The pupil should sit erect with the weight equally borne by both buttocks; the legs should be straight before the trunk, and the feet firmly resting on the floor. The book should be held about twelve inches from the eyes.

Spinal Curvatures.— It should be distinctly borne in mind that lateral curvature of the spine is a distortion of growth. The deformity appears and is developed during the growing years. It is more common in girls than in boys, for two reasons: that at the age when lateral curvature is first seen, girls grow more rapidly than boys; and their muscular system is less well developed.

In most early cases the faulty attitudes are clearly the result of muscular weakness. The growth in size has not been accompanied by a corresponding development of the muscles. This condition is most frequently met with in rapidly growing girls, and it is one of the most common causes of lateral curvature. In these cases proper gymnastics are indicated, but they should be prescribed and carried out with much care.

It is upon the erectness, suppleness, and strength of the spinal column that most of the power and grace of the body depend.

Lack of ventilation is a fertile cause of headache, anemia (or an impoverished condition of the blood in iron and oxygen), and dyspepsia. All these are rare before but common after twelve years of age.

Exercise.— In physical culture the object aimed at should be the symmetrical development of all the muscles of the body. Hence the necessity for bringing every individual muscle into play, at first for its development, and later for its maintenance.

The tendency of almost all forms of exercise is to develop some portion of the body at the expense of the rest. The most perfect form of exercise is therefore that one which will most nearly call into play all the muscles of the body.

Walking.— Walking is the only form of exercise which may be said to be universal. In walking the muscles of the chest get little exercise, and those of the spine and abdomen even less. In walking the arms should swing easily at the sides, both from a physiological and an esthetic point of view. If the girl is weak or is unaccustomed to take any exercise, the guide for the amount of exercise taken at any one time must be this: At the first sense of fatigue, stop at once and rest, otherwise positive harm instead of good may be accomplished. The girl who depends on walking for her outdoor exercise should walk at least three miles every day, and walk at the rate of three miles an hour.

After acquiring as great a walking speed as is consistent with a graceful and easy carriage, the running exercise should be begun, gradually increasing the distance, but not the rate of speed.

In exercising, all tight clothing about the neck, chest, and waist must be removed. Pure air and full breathing are required during and after exercise. Full breathing not only promotes the change of air in the lungs, but also quickens the functions of the circulation and digestion. Eating must be avoided shortly before or shortly after any considerable exercise, as it impairs digestion.

Running.— Running is the best exercise for developing the breathing capacity. While brisk walking is allowable, fast running is not. The rule for running is to begin slowly, run moderately for perhaps fifty feet, then increase the speed gradually; but in running for exercise, never speed to the utmost. A five-mile gait is quite sufficient. The run should be closed with the same moderation with which it was begun, and the girl should never stop short, as this sudden arrest of action gives a most undesirable shock to the heart.

In beginning to take any form of exercise the intensity and duration of the movements practiced must be increased very gradually, or positive harm instead of good will be done. As soon as fatigue is appreciable, the exercise should be discontinued and at once be followed by complete rest. Rapid respiration, palpitation or dizziness, headache, the face becoming pale or pinched or flushing suddenly, a feeling of great heat or excessive perspiration, are all danger signals showing that the exercise has already been carried too far and should cease at once. Continued over-exertion carried to a point of exhaustion leads to an obstinate irritability of the heart as well as to organic lesions.

Mountain-climbing, rowing, and bicycling call into play almost all the muscles of the body. Of all the outdoor exercises for girls, swimming is one of the most perfect. It not only calls into vigorous action most of the muscles of the body, but spares many of those muscles that are so commonly overworked, the most of the work being performed by muscles that are so little used as to have become flabby and weak.

Swimming and sea-bathing must be avoided by girls who have weak hearts and in whom the reaction after a plunge into cold water is never established; also by girls with heart disease or kidney disease.

The principal outdoor games are croquet, archery, golf, tennis, cricket, foot-ball, and base-ball. Of these, croquet is the mildest, and is for that reason a good beginning exercise. Croquet, archery, golf, and tennis are all defective in that they cause a greater development of the right than of the left side of the body.

As the greater majority of these outdoor exercises can only be indulged in for seven months of the year, they should be supplemented by exercises in the gymnasium for the remaining five winter months.

There should be the greatest variety possible in the kinds of exercise taken, not only to develop the body symmetrically, so as to obtain strength, vigor, grace, celerity, and accuracy of movement, but also because there is no such potent cause of fatigue as monotonous repetition of the same act, whether physical or mental.

It has been repeatedly proven that physical deterioration can be overcome by exercise, and that by so doing the mental capacity is greatly increased.

CHAPTER III.

ANATOMY OF THE GENERATIVE ORGANS.

The Vulva; the Hymen; Condition, of the Hymen as a Proof of Virginity; the Bladder; Vagina; Uterus; Respiratory Movements of the Uterus; Fallopian Tubes; Ovaries.

> "He that respects himself is safe from others;
> He wears a coat of mail that none can pierce."
>
> — LONGFELLOW.

The Vulva.— The female generative organs consist of three groups — the external, the intermediate, and the internal. The vulva, or external generative organs, comprises all those organs which are external to the body.

The vulva is pierced by two openings, the smallest and most anterior of which is the external opening of the urethra, or excretory duct of the bladder. This opening is surrounded by a slight eminence and has a somewhat puckered aspect.

The larger opening is the vaginal orifice. In the virgin this is partially closed by the hymen. About one inch back of this is the anus, or the external orifice of the large bowel. This part of the bowel is known as the rectum.

The Hymen.— The hymen consists of a thin duplicature of mucous membrane strengthened by fibrous tissue, and is stretched across the posterior part of the vaginal orifice, which it partly occludes. Rupture of the hymen usually, but not always, occurs during the first sexual intercourse. In rare cases it is found intact at the time of the birth of the first child. In women who have borne children the vaginal orifice is surrounded by small irregular elevations; these are the remains of the ruptured hymen, but are usually present only after labor has taken place, since the torn hymen is converted into eminences as the result of the pressure incident to childbearing, and not to coitus.

The Condition of the Hymen as a Proof of Virginity.— Formerly much stress was laid on the condition of the hymen as a proof of virginity. The hymen tightly closed, barely admitting the tip of a small index-finger, is positive evidence of virginity. But the hymen may lose its tone by a local catarrhal condition or by a general muscular relaxation; it may then become so relaxed that the only positive evidence rendered by the intact hymen is that the woman has not borne a child.

In a paper on the preservation of the hymen, Dr. Hannah M. Thompson writes: "Further, if the hymen was intended as a guarantee of moral character, and for moral protection, either of man or woman, would we not have some reason for reflecting on the wisdom and righteousness of a Creator who has failed to make equal provision, and to give a like guarantee of an uncorrupted manhood? As physicians, we know too well that where one woman enters the marriage relation tainted in body there are thousands of men reeking with disease; and there is no demonstrable test to distinguish these, no proof for the young woman of the virginity or virtue of the young man."

The Bladder.— The female bladder is relatively broad and capacious, and is also highly distensible. When the bladder is allowed to become overdistended, it is carried backward and tends to cause a backward displacement of the uterus. The urethra, or excretory duct of the bladder, is about an inch and a half long, and lies firmly imbedded in the anterior vaginal wall.

The Vagina.— The intermediate organ is the vagina. This is a musculo-membranous canal which connects the external with the internal organs of generation. The vagina lies in relation with the bladder and the urethra in front, and with the rectum behind. The vagina is sufficiently distensible to allow of the passage of so large a body as the child.

The Uterus.— The internal organs of generation are the uterus, the ovaries, and the Fallopian tubes. Of these, the ovaries and the uterus are the essential female organs of generation. The virgin uterus is a small, hollow, muscular organ, somewhat pear-shaped, whose cavity is about one and a half inches deep. The uterus is divided by a natural constriction into a body and a neck. The neck, or cervix, is somewhat spindle-shaped, and has a canal running through its center which opens by a small aperture — the so-called external orifice, — into the vagina. In the virgin uterus the apposition of the anterior and posterior walls reduces the cavity to little more than a longitudinal cleft. With the advent of old age the whole organ suffers marked atrophy.

The uterus is situated in the middle of the pelvic cavity, between the bladder and the lower bowel. It is held in place by broad elastic bands which go to different sides of the pelvis; it is also in part supported by the structures below and above it. But so loosely is the uterus held that it is easily pushed about — as, for instance, by a full bladder or a packed bowel. And persistently allowing the bladder to become overfull, and failure to have a daily evacuation of the bowels, are prolific sources of displacements of the womb.

Respiratory Movements of the Uterus. — When no constrictions are placed about the waist, the uterus moves freely up and down with every respiration. So distinctly and with such regularity do these movements take place that an operator by watching the movements of the uterus can tell the effect that the anesthetic is having on the patient's breathing. These so-called respiratory movements play a very important role in the circulation of the uterus, and in the return of the venous blood to the heart.

Anything which interferes with these movements, as the use of corsets, or of tight bands around the waist, prevents the free return of the venous blood. The uterus becomes congested, and through the constant abnormal weight of the organ itself, as well as the pressing down upon it from above of the superincumbent organs, the uterus is pushed down below its normal position, the ligaments whose duty it is to hold it up become relaxed, and the unhappy woman suffers all the agonies that are attendant on the "falling of the womb." For this reason the disorder is frequently met with in women who have never borne children as well as in those who have.

The Fallopian Tubes.— The Fallopian tubes extend from the upper, rounded angles of the uterus, within and along the free margin of the broad ligaments, for a distance of about two inches, to the vicinity of the ovaries, where each one terminates in a funnel-shaped orifice surrounded by a series of fringed processes. The lumen of the tube is narrowest at its inner end, where it opens into the cavity of the uterus by a minute orifice which scarcely admits a bristle; the diameter of the canal gradually increases until it reaches its ovarian extremity. The mucous lining of the tube is clothed by a single layer of hair-like epithelium, whose current sweeps from the ovarian toward the uterine end of the tube; and it is these movements which propel the ovum from the ovary to the uterus.

The Ovaries.— The ovaries are two small bodies of an almond shape, and lie on either side of the uterus. The bulk of the entire organ consists of connective tissue, in which lie imbedded the Graafian follicles or ovisacs, in which the ova are contained. These follicles or ovisacs are minute cells which are packed immediately beneath the surface, where they occur in all stages of development. With the increase in size which accompanies their development the follicles pass toward the surface, where they form a distinct projection, and at this point will occur the final rupture of the sac and the escape of the ovum. It is supposed that the ovum is grasped by the fringe-like extremity of the Fallopian tube and is carried through it by the movements of the ciliary epithelium to the uterus.

The formation of new follicles continues only for a short time after birth, when the Graafian follicles are the most numerous; the entire number contained within the ovaries of the child being estimated at over 70,000. In view of the unquestionably large number of follicles in very young ovaries, and the relatively small number of ova which reach maturity, the degeneration of many follicles after reaching a certain degree of development seems certain.

CHAPTER IV.

PHYSIOLOGY OF THE FEMALE GENERATIVE ORGANS.

Ovulation; Etiology of Menstruation; Uterine Nerve-supply; the Function of the Uterus; Stages of the Menstrual Cycle; Average

Duration of the Menstrual Flow; Character of tahe Flow; Relation of Ovulation to Menstruation; the Menstrual Wave; Definition of Menstruation; Premomitory Symptoms of the Flow; Hygiene of Menstruution.

> "Toil and grow strong; by toil the flaccid nerves
> Grow firm, and gain a more compacted tone."
>
> — ARMSTRONG.

Ovulation.— At birth the formation of the ova is nearly completed; the production of new cells probably ceases after the second year. The ovaries of the child of two years contain, therefore, the full quota of ova, although the vast majority of these cells always remain immature and undeveloped. While it is probable that a variable number of the immature ova undergo partial development before puberty, yet the advent of sexual maturity at that time marks the establishment of the regular development of the Graafian follicles and their contained ova, accompanied by the attendant phenomena of menstruation.

During the entire child-bearing period, or from about the age of fifteen to forty-five years, the development of the Graafian follicles and the discharge of the ova are continually taking place. The liberation of the ova usually takes place at definite times, which in general coincide with the menstrual epochs, one or more ova being set free at each period; but this is by no means invariable.

The ripe human ovum or germ cell is a spheric cell, about 0.2 mm. in diameter, consisting of granular protoplasm, in which lies a nucleus which contains the germinal spot. The proper cell-wall is a structure of great delicacy, outside of which is a secondary envelope.

Menstruation.— The etiology of menstruation has been variously explained at different epochs. The chief theories have been that of plethora, and the ovulation, the tubal, and the nerve theories.

First, the Theory of Plethora.— From the time of Hippocrates to 1835 the theory prevailed that in the female body the formation of blood is sufficiently rich to provide every four weeks for an overflow of the same, the evacuation of which becomes a necessity. It was believed that this excess of blood depended on an excess of formative power in the woman.

Second, the Ovulation Theory. — This was distinctly formulated about 1845. It construed the menstrual hemorrhage as a subsidiary phenomenon, entirely dependent on the periodic dehiscence of ovules. The changes supposed to take place in the Graafian follicles at each menstrual period were believed to involve a peculiar expenditure of nerve force, which was so much dead loss to the individual life of the woman. The growth of the Graafian vesicle and its contained ovum was supposed to cause an irritation of the nerves of the ovary, which was reflected to the entire nervous system. The gradual accumulation of this irritation finally caused a reflex action which determined an afflux of blood to the uterus and ovaries, which constitutes the catamenial flow.

The ovulation theory was refuted by the following facts: Ovulation may and does occur without menstruation; women who have never menstruated may conceive; conception may occur during lactation, without the menses having returned since the last parturition; children at birth have many ovules contained within the ovaries; ovulation may persist for a time after the menopause, and even pregnancy has occurred, although very rarely after this time; the menses may continue regularly after the removal of the ovaries and Fallopian tubes; this is exceptional, and, as a rule, the periods only continue for two or three years at longest.

Third, the Tubal Theory. — Lawson Tait thought that thorough removal of the tubes was far more essential in determining the menopause, and that cases of periodically recurring hemorrhage after the removal of the ovaries were to be explained by the fact that the tubes had not been sufficiently removed. As an anatomic and surgical fact, the tubes can never be wholly excised unless the upper part of the uterus is also amputated.

Fourth, the Nerve Theory of Menstruation. — This is based upon the following views:

1. That menstruation is a process directly controlled by a nerve-center situated in the lumbar region of the spinal cord.

2. That the menstrual impulses reach the uterus through two sets of nerves.

3. That menstruation is the result of nerve irritation, vascular congestion, and the subsequent relief of these by hemorrhagic discharges.

4. That hemorrhage from the uterus is the result either of a local uterine condition, or of influences outside of the uterus acting directly on the center.

5. That the removal of the appendages arrests menstruation by preventing the propagation of uterine influences to the center.

Uterine Nerve Supply.— One set of nerves causes contraction of the muscular fibers of the uterus, while the other set transmits impulses which bring about its vascular engorgement; and they are probably concerned in bringing about the determination of blood to the uterus and its appendages, which is so marked a feature of the menstrual process.

As the result of long-continued investigation, Johnstone has come to the conclusion that the lining membrane of the uterus belongs to that class of organs whose function it is to replace organic waste. "Menstruation is a periodic wasting away of those corpuscles that are too old to make a placenta." He has further found that, as compared with the uteri of very many of the lower animals, the human uterus is very scantily supplied with lymphatics, and the only way to rid the uterus of the overripe, and therefore consequently useless, tissue is to wash it out through the vagina by a blood-stream. The tough wall of the human uterus and the increased blood-pressure caused by the erect position cause the difference between menstruation in the human female and rut in the lower animals.

The strong light of recent investigations has necessitated the laying aside of many time-honored theories; and as the close of the nineteenth century has seen the emancipation of the uterus from the thralldom of the ovary, so we may believe that the twentieth century will find women of such fine physique as to prove the error of the popular fallacy that the cause of woman's weakness lies in the performance of her functions.

The Function of the Uterus.— The function of the uterus is to provide a favorable place for the reception of the product of conception, where it may be protected and nourished during the period of its development. The purpose of menstruation is to keep the uterus in suitable condition for the reception of this product of conception at any time. It is now known that the menstrual flow is not the whole of menstruation, and that the changes going on in the uterus are almost as continuous as the process of digestion. The whole of the reproductive life of woman has been divided into cycles of twenty-eight days each; these cycles have been divided into four stages.

Stages of the Menstrual Cycle.— The first or constructive stage is one of preparation for the reception of the ovum. During this stage the preparing of a decidua takes place, or building a nest for the expected egg; there is a swelling of the mucous membrane, an enlargement of the uterine glands, and an increase in the connective tissue. It is thought that this stage lasts for one week; when pregnancy does not occur, it is followed by degenerative changes.

The second or destructive stage is marked by destructive changes which give rise to the usual phenomena of the menstrual period; there is a discharge of blood, mucus, and disintegrated mucous membrane. The actively growing cells of the uterine lining membrane undergo rapid destructive changes, the fabric of the half-formed decidua tumbles to pieces, the turgid capillaries burst and pour out the menstrual flow, which sweeps away all the useless debris. The irritation sets up reflex uterine contractions, and so the blood is squeezed out of the distended capillaries and washes away the degenerated cells.

The third or reparative stage, as its name indicates, is one of repair, in which by constructive changes the epithelial lining which was thrown off is replaced by new, which is formed in from three to four days.

The fourth or quiescent stage includes the remaining twelve or fourteen days of the menstrual cycle, and represents the quiescent period prior to the initiative changes which mark the beginning of the next period.

Average Duration of the Menstrual Flow.— The average duration of the menstrual flow is five days, although the variations are considerable in healthy women. A flow lasting any place from two to six days is perfectly consistent with health; but a flow continuing less than two or more than six days generally indicates local or general disease.

Character of the Menstrual Flow.— For the first few hours, or perhaps for the first day, the flow is usually slight in quantity and light in color; on the second and third days the flow reaches its height, and is profuse and dark, but it should never be clotted; after this it gradually ceases. The amount of the flow varies from five to ten ounces. If less than five or six or more than eighteen napkins are pretty well saturated through, the amount may be considered abnormal.

Relation of Ovulation to Menstruation.— It has not yet been decided just in what relation the processes of ovulation and menstruation stand to each other. It is supposed that the transit of the ovum to the uterus occupies at least one week. It has been thought that the decidua of a particular menstrual period is related, not to the ovum discharged at that period, but to the ovum discharged at the preceding period.

The menstrual wave, or the wave of "supplementary nutrition,"[*] upon which the menstrual process ultimately depends, was first established by Dr. Mary Putnam Jacobi in the Boylston prize essay for 1876; showing that menstrual life is associated with a wave of well-marked vital energy, which manifests itself in a monthly fluctuation of the tempera ture of the body, in the daily amount of the excretion of urea and of carbonic acid, and of the rate and tension of the pulse. The wave attains its maximum during the week preceding menstruation, and slowly falls to its minimum, which is reached the week after menstruation.

* Dr. Goodman and Dr. Stephenson have since written on this subject, and the "wave" is often known as the Stephenson wave.

This wave indicates a periodic variation in the bodily metabolism, and is probably directly influenced by the rhythmic activity of the menstrual center. This observation would seem to be nullified by the fact that the phenomena referred to have been found to occur in men as well as in women; and that the lower animals also seem to show the same periodic variations. "It is therefore evident that the phenomena belong not to the function of menstruation, but to a general law of vital energy."

Definition of Menstruation.— Menstruation may, then, be defined as the periodic discharge of blood from the uterus, accompanied by the shedding of the epithelium of the body, as well as that of the uterine glands near their orifices.

The sanguineous discharge is due partly to the oozing of blood from the surfaces denuded of epithelium, and partly to active congestion. The discharge from the uterus is largely augmented by mucus secreted in increased quantity at this period from the enlarged uterine glands.

The tubes take some part in the process of menstruation; their mucous membrane is swollen, the epithelium is shed in places, and they are filled with a thin bloody fiuid, containing blood-corpuscles and cast-off epithelium cells.

The menstrual wave continues from puberty to the menopause; it is a nervous phenomenon. Ovulation is a progressive, non-periodic process; it begins before birth and continues till the ovarian tissue is atrophied or worn out.

Premonitory Symptoms of the Flow.— The premonitory symptoms of the monthly flow should not be so marked as to cause the individual any discomfort. The first indication of the return of the period should be the appearance of the flow. There is generally a feeling of abdominal fulness with some lassitude, and sometimes slight headache. The temperature is lower and the pulse is slower than at other times. This lowered tone of the system is an additional reason for increased care against exposure in wet or cold weather.

Hygiene of Menstruation.— During the menstrual periods all *cold baths* must be strictly prohibited, whether tub-baths or cold sponges. The reason of this is that the application of cold to the surface causes a driving in of the blood from the exterior of the body to the internal organs; and at the menstrual periods there is already a congested condition of the pelvic organs, and it must be remembered that congestion is the first stage of inflammation.

Hot or *warm sponge-baths* may be taken throughout the period; and the vulva should be bathed with warm water twice a day through the entire period of the flow, as this not only removes the clotted blood before it decomposes and becomes the source of irritation, but also removes other irritating matters, and prevents the nervousness that is caused by a local irritation.

It is strange how women who are scrupulously neat in all other respects will allow the smegma to collect in and about the vulva; as a matter of fact, for the purpose of cleanliness it is much more necessary that the external genitals should be washed twice a day with soap and water all through life than that the face should be washed that often.

Another question which is still *sub judice* is the necessity for and the frequency with which vaginal douches should be taken; all physicians are agreed that a vaginal douche taken immediately after the menstrual period is beneficial, as it removes all the debris of the flow, which is sometimes very irritating.

Exercise. – A moderate amount of exercise should be taken every day; this is needed now quite as much as at any other time, and only good can result from it. And no harm comes of a woman going out in the rain or in cold weather; as has been shown, the menstrual process is going on for a large part of the time, and the flow is only the external appearance, but during the time of the flow the woman must be unusually careful not to get her feet wet or to sit down with damp clothing on. Violent exercise of all kinds is to be prohibited at this time, as dancing, rides on the bicycle, gymnastics, and walks of over three miles. The reason for this is very obvious; the uterus has now reached the height of its turgescence, and is heavier than at any other time, hence the danger that displacements or a very profuse flow would be caused by any kind of violent exercise.

Treatment. – If the woman has been so unfortunate as to get caught out in a heavy rain so that her clothes have been wet through, or if in the cold weather she should come into the house thoroughly chilled, the best thing to do is to take off her wet things as quickly as possible, be well rubbed down with hot, rough towels, drink a cup of hot tea, go to bed at once and place a hot-water bag over the abdomen. She should remain in bed until the next morning, to the end that the circulation may regain its equilibrium as quickly as possible by the immediate relief of the pelvic congestion. If this exposure should have caused the sudden cessation of the flow, a hot mustard foot-bath should be taken. One tablespoonful of mustard is used to a gallon of water as hot as can be borne; the pail should be made as full as can be without running over, and a blanket wrapped around the pail and woman, so as to cause a profuse perspiration; this should be kept up for ten minutes; if the water cools off, hot water may be added.

CHAPTER V.

THE ANOMALIES OF MENSTRUATION.

Menorrhagia and Metrorrhagia; Dysmenorrhea; Amenorrhea; Leuchorrhea; Pruritus Vulvae.

> "Defer not till to-morrow to be wise,
> To-morrow's sun on thee may never rise."
>
> — CONGREVE

Menorrhagia and Metrorrhagia.— By menorrhagia is meant an excessive or too profuse menstrual flow; by metrorrhagia, a flow of blood between the menstrual periods. Neither one constitutes a disease by itself, but is a symptom of some pathologic condition.

It has already been stated that the excretory organs, by constantly eliminating from the system the worn-out material, keep the machine healthy and in good working order. Kept within natural limits, this elimination is the source of strength and health; beyond these limits, the menstrual flow becomes an actual hemorrhage that, by draining away the life, becomes the source of weakness and disease.

No physician would dare to bleed a man or woman once a month, year in and year out for thirty years; but, through ignorance or folly, this is what many girls do for themselves.

This excessive flow, aside from actual local disease, is brought about by excessive muscular exercise during menstruation; by the use of all stimulants, whether alcoholic beverages or quinin; as well as by the thinness of the blood.

When the flow is excessive, it must be considered a pathologic condition, which needs the physician's attention. Rest in the recumbent position is the first essential; the diet must be plain and unstimulating, and attention must be paid to the condition of the blood.

The general diseases which generally cause this condition are anemia, Bright's disease, malaria, the early stages of tuberculosis, and heart disease.

The local causes may be reflex, as powerful emotions; or due to local disease of the uterus and its appendages, as the various inflammations and displacements of the uterus, fibroid tumors, polypi, and cancer.

Dysmenorrhea is painful menstruation. The most frequent forms are due to uterine congestion; to mechanical causes, as a narrowing of the cervical canal, particularly at its internal opening, or to a constriction caused by the bending over of the uterus at the junction of the body and the neck; or to ovarian irritation.

The pain varies in intensity from slight discomfort to the most intense uterine colic, which is experienced in the lower part of the abdomen. In severe cases the general health becomes undermined, the nervous system gives way, and hysteria and other disorders of the nervous system result.

The congestive variety usually occurs in patients who have previously menstruated painlessly. The pain comes on suddenly with the flow and ceases when the flow stops; it is very severe and is generally accompanied by a diminution or a cessation of the flow. There is severe headache, marked diminution in the secretion of the kidneys, and general restlessness. The patient frequently experiences pain in walking, is easily fatigued, has leucorrhea and an irritable bladder.

In ovarian dysmenorrhea the pain precedes the flow for several days and ceases when a free flow is established. The pain is of a dull aching character, and may be felt on one or both sides of the abdomen, according as one or both ovaries are involved.

Amenorrhea.— In amenorrhea the menstrual flow may not appear for some years after it is normally due; or the flow may cease after some months or years of continuance; or the flow may be abnormally scanty or even absent.

The menstrual flow is much later in appearing in some families than in others, so that this may be considered as a family idiosyncrasy; and if the girl's health is good, it need cause no anxiety. If, on the contrary, the girl has severe headaches, or suffers in any way, the physician should be summoned at once, as the absence of menstruation may be indicative of some serious pathologic condition.

A scanty flow is often indicative of thinness of the blood; on the other hand, serious anemias often lead to profuse menorrhagias or metrorrhagias, as has already been stated. The cause of the profound anemia itself may be insufficient nutrition, overwork, or lack of exercise.

Scanty menstruation is often seen to occur in fevers, in the later stages of consumption, in advanced Bright's disease, in malaria, or in any other very serious disease. In these cases it seems to be a conservative process on the part of nature in the run-down state of the system. As consumption progresses menstruation generally ceases absolutely, never to return again; and in this case nothing should be done to try to induce a return of the flow.

Great shock sometimes causes a sudden cessation of the flow; and sometimes a sea-voyage, followed by the change of habitat, will cause an obstinate form of amenorrhea.

But it cannot be too well understood that, after the menstrual flow has been regularly established, it continues with the greatest regularity throughout the child-bearing period, unless the exposure to wet or cold has been sufficiently severe to cause great indisposition on the part of the woman. In this case it is possible that, if the exposure took place just previous to the time of the expected flow, one period may remain out. But except in case of serious illness,— as for example, typhoid fever,— two or more periods do not fail to appear except in the case of pregnancy.

Leucorrhea.— Leuchorrhea, or "whites," is a mucous or mucopurulent discharge from the vagina; it may be a symptom of uterine or vaginal disease.

Immediately after the menstrual flow there is a well-marked vaginal secretion which is whitish in appearance; it may be transparent or of a milky color, and is sometimes very acrid. This secretion may also precede the flow, and there is nothing abnormal in this. But any discharge occurring between the periods sufficient to stain the clothing— the so-called whites or leucorrhea— is abnormal, and is caused by an inflammation of the vagina or the neighboring parts. In addition to the discharge there is heat and swelling of the parts, more or less local distress, and generally intense nervousness.

If the disease is not cured, it may become chronic. The pain, heat, and scalding disappear, but a copious discharge continues, and in this stage the disease may be very obstinate and greatly reduces the strength. The constant drain breaks down the system, producing pallor, debility, pain in the back, palpitation, indigestion, and so forth.

The character of the discharge in leucorrhea varies considerably, from a whitish or mucous secretion, to a yellowish or mucopurulent secretion, and is debilitating in proportion as it is profuse. It is to be remembered that this is not in itself a disease, but indicates a disease of some of the pelvic organs; and that all such inflammations left to themselves incline to grow worse.

A severe leucorrhea is generally attended with frequent and finally painful micturition; pain in walking in the lower part of the abdomen, which may become so severe as to compel the patient to go to bed.

Pruritus Vulva.— This is an intense and persistent itching of the vulva, and is a symptom rather than a disease. It is not an infrequent result of leucorrhea, the acrid discharge of the latter leading to an irritation of the parts; this causes rubbing of the parts until a veritable inflammation is produced.

Other causes of pruritus vulvae are: The local congestion, such as occurs at the menstrual period, or in certain cases of pelvic inflammations, or in early pregnancy; constipation; sedentary habits; congestion of the liver; incontinence of urine, and diabetes. When dependent on the latter, the malady is most obstinate in yielding to treatment. Indigestible foods or drinks, the rubbing of the clothes, the friction of walking, and the heat of the bed act as exciting causes in those predisposed to it.

The essential treatment here is to at once ascertain and remove the cause; aids in the treatment are vaginal douches and cooling lotions.

CHAPTER VI.

THE MARRIAGE QUESTION.

Herbert Spencer's Definition of Love; What Constitutes a Suitable Husband; Best Age for Marriage; Shall Cousins Marry? Contraindications to Marriage; Do Reformed Profligates Make Good Husbands? the Proper Length of Time for the Engagement; the Right Time of the Year to Marry; the Selection of the Wedding Day.

> "Well, Brutus, thou art noble; yet, I see,
> Thy honourable mettle may be wrought
> From that it is disposed: Therefore, 'tis meet
> That noble minds keep ever with their likes.
> For who so firm that cannot be seduced?"
>
> — *"Julius Caesar."*

Herbert Spencer's Definition of Love.— "Love is habitually spoken of as though it were a simple feeling, whereas it is the most compound, and therefore the most powerful, of all the feelings. Added to the purely physical elements of it, are first to be noticed those highly complex impressions produced by physical beauty; around which are aggregated a variety of pleasurable ideas, not themselves amatory, but which have an organized relation to the amatory feelings. With this there is united the complex sentiment we term affection— a sentiment which, as it can exist between those of the same sex, must be regarded as an independent sentiment, but one which is here greatly exalted. Then there is the sentiment of admiration, respect, reverence, in itself one of considerable power, and which in this relation becomes in a high degree active. There comes next the feeling called the love of approbation. To be preferred above all the world, and that by the one admired above all others, is to have the love of approbation gratified in a degree passing every other experience, especially as there is added that indirect gratification of it which results from the preference being witnessed by others. Further, the allied emotion of self-esteem comes into play. To have succeeded in gaining such attachment from and sway over another is a proof of power which cannot fail to agreeably excite *amour propre*. Yet again, the proprietary feeling has its share in the general activity. There is the pleasure of possession, the two belonging to each other. Once more, the relation allows of an extended liberty of action. Toward each other a strained behavior is requisite. Around each there is a suitable boundary that may not be crossed; an individuality on which none may trespass. But in this case the barriers are thrown down, and the love of unrestrained activity is gratified. Finally, there is an exaltation of sympathies, egotistic pleasures of all kinds are doubled by another's sympathetic participation, and the pleasures of another are added to the egotistic pleasures. Thus around the physical feeling forming the nucleus of the whole, are gathered the feelings produced by personal beauty that constitutes simple attachments, of self-esteem, of property, of love of freedom, of sympathy. These, all greatly exalted and severally tending to reflect their excitements on one another, unite to form the mental state we call love. And as each of them is comprehensive of multidinous states of consciousness, we may say that this passion fans into immense aggregate most of the elementary excitations of which we are capable; and that hence results its irresistible power."

What Constitutes a Suitable Husband. — It is desirable that the husband shall be a few years older than the wife. Man is later in coming to maturity, and also retains his sexual powers considerably longer than woman; so that for these functions to cease about the same time, the wife must be younger than the husband. A difference of from two to five years is best; if the parties are young, it is not essential that the husband should be much the wife's senior, as it is later in life. The husband may be ten years older, but a greater disparity of age than this is rarely compatible with congeniality of tastes and dispositions, so essential to a happy married life. The woman who risks her happiness with a man many years younger than herself violates a precept of nature.

The average stature of the man is about three inches greater than that of the woman, and in the physiologic marriage any great deviation from this should be avoided.

The essentials for a happy marriage may be summed up as follows: that the parties shall be of suitable age; that they shall be physically well mated and in full sympathy with each other's views of life, of the same social position, and of equal education.

The Best Age for Marriage.— The reproductive life begins with puberty, but maturity is not reached before the age of twenty-one. It is only then that the standard of development is reached that is most compatible with the successful bearing of the grave responsibilities of wifehood and motherhood. The too early exercise of the reproductive functions leads to increased suffering on the part of the mother, depresses her vitality, and increases her liability to disease. Statistics show that the mortality is very much greater where girls marry under twenty years of age.

The offspring are apt to be small and ill developed, and die in large numbers in early life; only a small percentage live long and robust lives. In France it has been observed that where the fear of conscription has caused many young people to marry the offspring were lacking in vigor. Among the offspring of immature parents there is a larger proportion of idiots, cripples, criminals, scrofulous, insane, and tubercular than among the children of nubile parents.

In our climate women are best fitted to become wives and mothers between the ages of twenty-four and twenty-eight years. Before this age neither their self-knowledge, their knowledge of the world, nor their experience is sufficiently mature to fit them to wisely make the choice of a companion for life, or to become mothers. After forty, most women cannot hope for children. Men had better wait until between the ages of twenty-seven and thirty years, before they undertake the responsibilities of parenthood.

Shall Cousins Marry?— They might if both families were perfectly healthy; but as few families are without some lurking predisposition to disease, it is not well, as a rule, to run the risk of developing this by too repeated unions.

Contraindications to Marriage.— Young women in whose family there is a distinct history of such hereditary diseases as cancer, tuberculosis, or insanity for two generations back, should not marry at all. Not only is this a fearful legacy to hand down to their children, but pregnancy and child-bearing very decidedly favor the development of these diseases.

Syphilis in either sex is a distinct bar to marriage; first, the party married is sure to contract the disease, even though it may have been supposed to have been cured. Fortunately, the children of such marriages are generally still-born; still, they do sometimes live, and are most pitiable and sickly objects. For any one to marry under these conditions is a crime against society, against the State, and against posterity.

Women who have serious forms of heart disease, tuberculosis, or Bright's disease would, by becoming pregnant, run a serious risk of losing their lives toward the close of the pregnancy or at the time of their confinement. In case of heart disease, the pulmonary congestion that accompanies pregnancy, together with the encroachment of the pregnant uterus on the cavity of the chest, would greatly add to the embarrassment of the heart's action.

In normal pregnancy there is some congestion of the kidneys; where there is actual disease of the kidneys prior to the pregnancy, this congestion is apt to become so severe as to threaten the woman's life. These organic diseases are not to be confounded with functional diseases which are dependent on some other cause; as palpitation of the heart due to indigestion, or heart murmurs dependent on the thin state of the blood, or congestion of the kidneys due to exposure to cold;— all of which may be cured by proper treatment.

Should a woman with a fibroid tumor marry, she would run a great risk to her life; she should have the tumor removed, or, if this is not possible, she should give up all thoughts of marriage, since the increased irritation and congestion consequent upon the marital relations would tend to favor its growth. Should pregnancy ensue, delivery might be attended with serious complications, as very difficult labor, postpartum hemorrhage, or, as these tumors have but little vitality, and the pressure to which they are subjected during labor is liable to cause their death, disorganization, sloughing, and, as a result, puerperal septicemia.

Sometimes there is such a lack of development of the genital organs as to prevent the woman from having children.

Two persons with even a slight tendency to the same disease, either inherited or acquired, should not intermarry, even if they are in comparatively good health at the time. Their offspring would be quite sure to inherit their diseased tendencies.

Persons whose constitutions have been somewhat injured, but who are not tainted with actual disease, may rear children much healthier than themselves, provided their own lives are wisely regulated. If they are growing better all the time, and are not too much broken in constitution, it may be safe for them to marry.

Among the Jews the physician is frequently consulted before matrimonial alliances are contracted. This custom could not but be of universal benefit; many local or general diseases would be eradicated before marriage, and in this way much suffering and unhappiness would be spared; or, in other cases, the patient would be advised of the inadvisability of marriage.

Do Reformed Profligates Make Good Husbands?— The manner of life that has been led by this class of men is such as to undermine their health, if not to have rendered them physical wrecks. There is the overindulgence in alcoholic beverages, and perhaps, added to this, some drug habit. In addition to this, these men early in their career are apt to become infected with some of the venereal diseases, or perhaps with all of them— gonorrhea, syphilis, and so forth; and these diseases have the horrible characteristics of becoming latent. A man who contracts this kind of a disease can never be really sure that he is cured. All venereal diseases are highly contagious.

It is now a well-established fact that gonnorrheal infection is not only one of the most common causes of pelvic inflammations in women, but that these same inflammations are of the most virulent types, unless they are recognized and treated in the early stages. It is also a well-known fact that a large percentage of married women suffer from this disease. Sterility almost always results.

In the case of a syphilitic parent, one or two children may be born, but the offspring is generally sickly and diseased. Inebriety as well as sexual excesses are both well recognized as distinct forms of disease accompanied by degeneracy of brain tissue. It is nothing less than criminal for such men to have children, since these children would at least inherit the tendency to the same diseases, if they did not actually have them; there is also a strong probability of such children being born idiots or imbeciles.

It is therefore self-evident that, instead of a reformed profligate making a good husband, he must make a very diseased one. It has therefore been suggested that the parents of the prospective bride should demand from the intended groom a certificate of freedom from all venereal diseases by a physician of their own selection. Also that there should be legislation upon the subject, and that before a man is granted a license of marriage, he should have a certificate from the health officer of freedom from syphilis, gonorrhea, and tuberculosis.

The Proper Length of Time for the Engagement.— A period not shorter than three months, nor longer than one year, should elapse between the engagement and the marriage.

There are strong physiologic reasons against long engagements: they keep the affections and the passions in an excited and unnatural condition, which after a time tends to weaken the nervous system and undermine the health. These evil consequences are common to both sexes. It is far better that the subject of marriage should not be entertained at all unless the circumstances are such that the union might with propriety be effected at once.

The Right Time of the Year to Marry.— When woman marries she enters upon a new life, and a very trying one. Extreme heat and extreme cold are both very taxing to the human economy. Midsummer and midwinter are therefore both objectionable, but especially the former.

The Selection of the Wedding-day.— This is by common consent left to the bride. She should select a time about ten or fifteen days after the end of one of her menstrual periods, as this is the time of comparative sterility, and it is most desirable that the first sexual relations should be fruitless.

PART II.— MARRIAGE.

CHAPTER VII.

THE ETHICS OF MARRIED LIFE.

The Wedding Journey; the Ethics of Married Life; Shall Husband and Wife Occupy the Same Bed? the Comsummation of Marriage; the Marital Relation; Times when Marital Relations Should be Suspended.

> "If it is possible to perfect mankind, the means of doing so will be found in the medical sciences."— DESCARTES.

The Wedding-journey.— The wedding-journey, which was formerly the cause of so much discomfort to both husband and wife, has fortunately gone out of vogue; and in its place has come the retirement to a quiet country or seaside spot, away from the prying eyes of friends. Thus the nervous strain incident to sight-seeing and travel is avoided.

The Ethics of Married Life.— It has been said that God set men and women in pairs in order that they might perfect each other and complete each other's happiness. The secret of all true happiness in life lies in the spirit of altruism; one must be able to wholly forget herself and to find her happiness in the welfare of others.

The woman who exhausts herself physically and financially on the preparation of her trousseau and her wedding does her husband a wrong by bringing him a wife who is on the verge of nervous prostration.

The secret of a happy married life depends to no small extent on the very beginning: the relation is so entirely new, and much lies hidden in the character of each that was never suspected by the other.

Between husband and wife there must always be mutual concessions, forbearance, and sympathy; a mutual helpfulness to attain all that is best. This, of course, implies that the life of each is an open book for the other to read; that there is an unreserved exchange of thought; and that no privilege is claimed by the one that would not willingly be accorded to the other.

"How many men," says Balzac, "proceed with women as the monkey of Cassan with the violin; they have broken the heart without knowing it, as they have tarnished and disdained the jewel whose secret they never understood. Almost all men are married in ignorance of women and of love. They have commenced by forcing open the doors of a strange house and have wished to be well received in its salon. But the most ordinary artist knows that there exists between him and his instrument— his instrument which is made of wood or ivory— a sort of indefinable friendship. He knows by experience that it has taken years to establish this mysterious rapport between an inert material and himself. He could not have divined at the first stroke all its resources and caprices, its faults and its virtues. His instrument only became a soul for him and a source of melody after long study; he only came to understand it as two friends after the most learned interrogation.

"So the world is full of young women who grow pale and feeble, sick and suffering. The ones are a prey to inflammations more or less severe; the others remain under the dominion of nervous attacks more or less violent. All these husbands have caused their own unhappiness and ruin. Never begin married life with a rape. To demand of a young girl whom one has seen forty times in fifteen days to love you because of the law, the king, and justice is an absurdity.

"Love is the union of necessity and of sentiment. Happiness in marriage is the result of perfect understanding between the spirits of husband and wife. From this it happens that in order to be happy, a man is obliged to bind himself to certain rules of delicacy and honor. After taking advantage of the social laws which consecrate the necessity, it is necessary to obey the secret laws of nature, in order to make the sentiments flourish. If a man places his happiness on being loved, it is necessary that he should love sincerely; nothing resists a veritable passion."

Shall Husband and Wife Occupy the Same Bed?— Among civilized nations custom differs in this regard; in Germany, for instance, the husband and wife occupy separate beds in the same room; formerly in this country it was almost the universal custom for husband and wife to occupy the same bed. The current of opinion has changed in this respect, and it is now considered in the highest interests of both that they shall occupy not only separate beds, but separate rooms; these rooms communicating through a door which connects their respective dressing-rooms. This is unquestionably the best arrangement from the hygienic as well as from the ethical point of view. Health requires that one-third of the time shall be spent in sleep; the bed was made for sleep; and the most refreshing sleep can only be obtained by occupying the bed alone. If two persons occupy the same bed and one is restless, the sleep of the other is necessarily disturbed. Again, two persons occupying the same bed necessitates the same hour for rising and retiring, which is not always convenient or agreeable. Balzac writes on this subject: "To put the system of separate bed-rooms into practice is to attain to the highest degree of intellectual power and of virility. By what syllogism man arrived at establishing as a custom that of man and wife sleeping together, a practice so fatal to happiness, to health, to pleasure, and even to self-love, would be curious to seek out." If for financial reasons it is not possible to have separate bed-rooms, the German custom of having separate beds should be adopted.

The Consummation of Marriage.— The consummation of marriage is often attended with difficulty owing to the rigidity of the hymen; this, if present, must usually be ruptured before connection takes place. Great gentleness and care must be exercised by the husband if it does not readily yield, the use of hot vaginal injections should be kept up for several weeks before the trial is repeated. These usually relax the parts very considerably; but if coitus is still found impossible, it is better to consult a physician at once, when a simple operation will generally remove the trouble and the woman is spared much suffering. In no case is any violence on the part of the husband allowable, as it might produce irreparable injuries.

There is always more or less suffering on the part of the wife at first, partly due to the rupture of the hymen, and partly to the forcible dilatation of the vagina and she should be allowed a sufficient time for nature to repair these injuries. By so doing, the constitutional disturbances and the nervous disorders which are so very prevalent may be prevented. Too frequent indulgence at this period is a prolific source of inflammatory diseases, and often occasions sterility and ill-health.

The first nuptial relations should be fruitless, in order that any indisposition arising therefrom should have had time to disappear before the woman becomes pregnant.

The Marital Relation.— It is most important for the interest of both parties that there should be chastity in the marriage relation as well as out of it. Many young couples have had their lives ruined by excessive sexual indulgence. The effect is usually most severe upon the husband, yet the wife becomes weak, nervous, and excitable. Sexual excess is also the grave of domestic affection. The general rule given is that coitus should never take place oftener than every seven or ten days. When coitus is succeeded by langour, depression, or malaise, it has been indulged in too frequently.

Among civilized people there are three widely diferent views as to the proper course to be pursued:

First, those who maintain that sexual intercourse should not take place except for the propagation of the species.

Second, those who believe that the act is a love relation, mutually demanded and enjoyed by both sexes, and serving other purposes besides that of procreation.

Third, those who hold that sexual intercourse is a physical necessity for the man, but not for the woman.

The first theory, "that the sexual relations should never be sustained save for the purpose of procreation," has many advocates. They teach that there are other uses for the procreative element than the generation of offspring, and far better uses than its waste in pleasures. They claim that a life of total chastity increases the physical and mental vigor; and there will result a procreation on the mental and spiritual planes, instead of on the physical ones.

They also claim that to woman belongs the creative power; that she must choose when a new life shall be evolved; and that only by adhering to this law can she be protected in the highest function of her being— the function of maternity.

The adherents of the second theory, "that the act is a love relation, mutually demanded and enjoyed by both sexes, and that it serves other purposes besides that of procreation," claim that the female sexual life indicates that the healthy woman is neither indifferent nor passive in the generative act. It has much the same effect as in man— a powerful increase in her sensations, whole groups of muscles are set in motion, and the uterus as well as the entire nervous system are in an excited condition and activity. And that it is the province of the mother to decide when a new life should begin.

The third theory, "that sexual intercourse is a physical necessity for the man, but not for the woman," is by far the most widely accepted. We will consider, first, the practical results of this last theory; and, second, the scientific basis on which it rests.

It is generally acknowledged that this practice has done more to cause domestic misery, sickness, and death than that dreadful scourge of the human race, tuberculosis.

This man, accustomed all his life to gratify his sexual passions promiscuously, marries a virtuous young girl. In her menstrual periods she has had to do only with the secondary phenomena; with the expulsion of the ova not at all. She has had no instruction in the corresponding physiologic life of the man, and is astonished at the male sexual indications, and is led to believe in their physiologic necessities. The result is that she not only suffers physically, but feels outraged and disgraced. She is liable to the chance of maternity at any time; and such offspring will probably be sickly.

Passion is presented to the young wife in so hideous a guise that it will take the utmost consideration of her husband afterward to enable her to completely overcome her repugnance. If she be worn and weary of excesses in the early days of her married life, the husband will have only himself to blame if he is bound all his life to an apathetic and irresponsive wife. Husbands place great strains upon the affections of their wives, and lower themselves almost past reinstatement in their respect and esteem.

Lastly, on what scientific basis does this "physilogic necessity" for sexual gratification on the part of the male rest? Analogy with the lower animals does not bear it out. Among animals, except in rare instances under domestication, the female admits the male in sexual embrace only for procreation. Among many savage tribes this same rule has but few exceptions. The analogies between the male and the female sexual organs; between seminal emissions and menstruation; between the sexual life of the male and of the female, only go to accentuate the fact that this so-called physiologic necessity on the part of the male has arisen chiefly through the difference of education; so that it has come to be that the woman is chaste and the man is degraded; that the woman is too sentimental and the man too passionate. From a purely medical standpoint, the most eminent physicians and physiologists of the day all unite in advocating a chaste and continent life, simply for the sake of the man's own health, independently of all other considerations.

Times when Marital Relations Should be Suspended.— The marital relations should always be suspended during the menstrual period. During pregnancy intercourse should never, or at least very rarely, be indulged in. At this time the mother needs to conserve all her strength and energies for herself and child; and any sexual relations during this time increase the sufferings of the mother and impair the vitality of the child. It has been even suggested that much of the pain during parturition would be avoided by entire continence during pregnancy. Intercourse during the early months of pregnancy is a frequent cause of abortion. Women who have supposed that they have never been pregnant have in reality been having abortions every second or third month.

A woman should never be subjected to coitus until three months after delivery. During lactation intercourse should never, or at least very rarely, be indulged in; as the function of lactation makes a heavy drain on the strength of the mother, and anything which would further weaken her would tend to impoverish the quality of the milk and thus the child would suffer.

CHAPTER VIII.

SEXUAL INSINCT IN WOMEN.

Sexual Instinct in Women; Excessive Coitus; Causes of Sexual Excitability.

> "Virtue, the strength and beauty of the soul,
> Is the best gift of heaven."
>
> — ARMSTRONG.

Sexual Instinct in Women.— After careful observation of the sexes in the married state, it is found that the sexual appetence is less in women than it is in men. Much of this difference in sexual appetence is doubtless due to the chastity of their lives, coupled with and resulting from the difference of education. The girl is taught repression, and the boy expression; that girls must be chaste; that chastity for boys is impossible.

According to the intensity of the sexual instinct women have been divided into three classes: A larger number than is supposed have little or no sexual feeling. Second, those who are subject to strong passion; this class is larger than the first, but small as compared with the whole of their sex. Third, those in whom the sexual appetite is moderate; this class comprises the vast majority of women.

And, even granting to woman more pleasure in sexual indulgence than usually comes to her by largest allowance, it is safe to say that in nine cases out of ten maternity, with its early pains and later cares, greatly lessens her power of enjoyment; and that for the larger part of her married life she is either positively distressed by the apparently necessary demands of her husband upon her, and irresponsive to them, or kept to a cheerful response by a self-abnegation and regard for his comfort, not to say fear of his moral aberration, which is a positive drain upon her health and strength.

Excessive Coitus.— Those who are most frequently found to suffer from venereal excesses are the newly married; especially if they have weak constitutions and excitable temperaments. A great deal of mischief is done by two persons of unequal constitutions being matched together; the husband may exhaust the wife or vice versa, the weaker party being constantly tempted to exceed their strength. In all sexual matters there must be a consideration for others. It is not so much from selfishness as from ignorance that such a mistake is made. The ignorance comes from a lamentable morbid delicacy which prevails on all sexual matters, and which prevents all open and rational conversation on them, even between those who have the most intimate knowledge of each other.

When the conjugal act is repeated too often, the man will become gradually conscious of diminished strength, diminished nerve force, and diminished mental powers. Excess weakens a man's energies, and enervates and effeminates him. Moreover, it renders him liable to an infinity of diseases and a readier victim to death.

Not only is the strength of the constitution lowered by the excessive expenditure of force and matter requisite for the perpetuation of the species, but this lowered standard of vitality is transmitted to children. There can be but little doubt that this is one of the reasons why so many healthy parents beget sickly children, who die early. They have exhausted themselves of the material from which a new life is created, and so it is not properly started at the beginning and never reaches its highest development. To the truth of this statement attests the mental imbecility, the pallid and attenuated forms, of the children who are the earlier products of marriage. The effect of excessive coitus in women is seen by the confirmed ill health of so many women after marriage and repeated child-bearing. A large number of these cases are dependent upon alteration and diseases of the genitalia; but a considerable number are unconnected with local disease, and in many other cases the health is never regained after all local phenomena have disappeared.

Sexual excitement in the woman causes certain congestion of the genital organs; and at the time of the orgasm there is a reflex movement which corresponds to erection, and which consists of a peristaltic movement of the tubes and uterus; to the uterus also is ascribed an act of suction by which the spermatozoa are drawn up into its interior. Even when pregnancy does not follow, the too frequent excitation and activity of the uterus in weak constitutions causes illness, first of the genital organs and then of the nervous system.

Local diseases caused in women by excessive coitus are: vaginal catarrh, acute catarrh of the vulva, acute inflammation of the lining membrane of the uterus as well as of the uterus itself, inflammation of the ovaries, and even peritonitis. It is also known to be an important factor in the origin of blood-tumors and of cancer of the uterus. Especially is coitus at a time of great physical fatigue liable to be provocative of uterine inflammations. Aside from ethical considerations, coitus during the menstrual period may be the cause of rupture of the impaired blood-vessels, thus causing blood-tumors. Excessive coitus is a well-known cause of chronic inflammation of the uterus; that is, a habitual congestion of the uterus is induced by excessive sexual intercourse. This has been frequently mentioned by authors as leading to enlargement of the uterus in the non-pregnant condition; and it is a still more potent factor in the recently impregnated organ, whose tissues are succulent and the vessels enlarged, a condition inviting congestion and enhancing the susceptibility to engorgement.

The general manifestations of impaired health in women due to excessive coitus are: chronic anemia, with malnutrition; impaired and altered functions in all the organs, especially those of the nervous system. Menorrhagia is apt to be induced by overstimulation of the ovaries, together with exhaustion and sexual apathy.

The source of so much misery is the increasing physical weakness of the female and the increasing nervous weakness of the male, with an increasing sexual excitability, two factors of tragic effect for the wife. Here is seen the unfortunate result of teaching two kinds of morals, one for men and another for women.

Causes of Sexual Excitability.— Too frequent genital irritation, onanism, too frequent intercourse, alcohol, too rich and too highly seasoned foods, lack of exercise.

Treatment of Sexual Excitability. — Avoid alcohol and precocious puberty. Strictest attention must be paid to the diet; everything is to be avoided which is difficult of digestion or which retards it. The following articles of diet must all be avoided: cheese, foods seasoned with pepper and curry, highly salted and acid foods, and all rich foods; and meat must be eaten only in moderate quantities. Constipation irritates the genitalia directly and increases the inflammation. The close relation of Venus and Bacchus is known not only in mythology. Carbonated waters are to be especially avoided, such as soda, seltzers, Preblauer, Geisshubler, and acid waters; also champagne and beer, heavy Italian, Spanish, and English wines. All alcoholic drinks must be forbidden.

As heavy gymnastics as the strength of the individual will admit, and plenty of exercise out-of-doors must be taken. There must also be constant mental and physical employment. In women sexual excitability is often caused by local diseases, and passes off with their cure; if not, she must use her will-power, and take the various forms of cold baths. Sexual intercourse not oftener than once in two or three weeks, and avoid all intimate approaches; if this is not sufficient, she will have to leave her husband for a few months.

CHAPTER IX.

STERILITY.

Sterility; the Prevention of Conception and the Limitation of Offspring; the Crime of Abortion; Infidelity in Women.

> "Never let yourselves do evil that good may come. If you do, you hinder the coming of the real, the perfect good in its due time."
>
> — PHILLIPS BROOKS.

Sterility.— Conception is least apt to take place from the tenth day after one period until the third day before the next; but there is practically no time during a woman's sexual life when she may not be impregnated; in this connection it must be remembered that the spermatozoa stay alive in her for more than a week.

During lactation women are generally sterile, especially in the first months which follow the accouchement, because the vital forces are then concentrated on the secretion of milk.

The age of the wife at the time of marriage has much to do with the expectation of children. As the age increases over twenty-five years the interval between the marriage and the birth of the first child is lengthened. For it has been ascertained that not only are women most fecund between twenty and twenty-five years, but that they begin their career of child-bearing sooner after marriage than either their younger or older sisters.

A wife who has had children and ceases to conceive for three years will probably bear no more.

When marriages are fruitless, the wife is almost always blamed; but it is by no means the wife that is always at fault; many husbands are absolutely sterile. Every man is not prolific who enjoys good health and is vigorous. Gross states that in one case out of six the sterility was due to the male. Kehrer, after a series of carefully conducted experiments, has arrived at the conclusion that in at least a third of the cases of sterile marriages the husband was the party at fault, and that gonorrhea was the cause of the barrenness.

Venereal diseases have their share of influence, and the gonorrheal infection is a potent cause of sterility. It is by no means proved that syphilis has any unfavorable influence on conception, though abortions due to this are frequent.

Gonorrhea often prevents conception by the inflammation traveling up the womb, and along the Fallopian tubes to the ovaries, whose covering is rendered thick and dense, so that the ovum cannot escape, or if it does, the fimbriated end of the tube is so agglutinated that it cannot grasp the ovum.

Alcoholism is considered a cause of sterility. It evidently does diminish the sexual potency in the male, and for this the female is often blamed.

It does not follow because a woman has not given birth to a child that she has not conceived. The life of an infant for a long time after birth is a frail one, and before birth its existence is extremely precarious; it often perishes a few days after conception. A period coming on a few days late, and at the same time one which is unusually profuse, is the only evidence which the young wife may have of an abortion. Among prostitutes, the frequent delay of menstruation, then abundant hemorrhage, is in many cases only habitual abortion, and leads to changes in the generative organs which must result in sterility. A tendency to miscarriage may therefore be all that stands in the way of having a family; this can frequently be remedied.

Sexual incompatibility is well known to exist; prominent examples being Augustus and Livia; Napoleon and Josephine. It is also a well-known fact that frigidity is a cause of barrenness. A short separation of husband and wife is often salutary in its influence upon fertility.

It is a well-established fact that the time immediately before the period, but still more that immediately following the period, are the most favorable times for conception to take place; the remaining quiet in bed of the woman after the generative act is also favorable to conception.

The most frequent causes of sterility in women are inflammation of the lining membrane of the uterus, or of the neck of the uterus, or of both. The source of this condition in women who have had children is most frequently due to parturition or abortion. In the newly married it may be due to a previously existing slight uterine catarrh in a displaced uterus, or it may be a manifestation of a run-down state of the system. In a majority of the newly married, however, the inflammation of the endometrium is probably due to the first efforts at conjugal approach. Many young women as the result of the preparation of the trosseau, augmented by a round of gaities at the time of marriage, enter the married state in a condition bordering on physical and nervous exhaustion; and then begin engorgements and inflammations which lead to future suffering and to sterility. Displacements and flexions of the uterus also cause sterility. Such displacements of the neck of the uterus may occur that, instead of lying in a pool of semen, as it should, it is above, in front of, or away from it, and this may prevent conception.

Vulvar and vaginal hyperesthesia, inflammations of the vulva, undue shortness of the vagina, unless great care is exercised by the husband, will induce painful coitus, and may bring about sterility by favoring the formation of a copulation sac outside of the axis of the uterine canal, and consequently misdirection of the semen.

Scrofula, probably by its effects on the general condition, leading to deficient development of the whole body, the genital organs included, may be productive of sterility.

The female being less passionate than the male, the orgasm comes on later with her, or the male orgasm occurs so soon that she may not reach that stage at all. If both were simultaneous, it is reasonable to suppose that conception would be more likely to occur.

Ovulation is doubtless more frequently performed in some women than in others. Some women conceive with more or less regularity every fifteen or eighteen months, and others at intervals of several years.

The effect of repeated coition, provided that impregnation does not take place at once, is to engorge the uterine vessels, to alter the nature of the glandular secretions, to cause profound reflex disturbances, and thus to produce such changes in the endometrium as to lead to local inflammation and to general nervous exhaustion. Backache, leucorrhea, and irritable bladder are the first symptoms of this disorder; but frequently there are added to these, headache, indigestion, rectal tenesmus, painful and profuse menstruation. In many cases the disease continues in a mild catarrhal form, giving the woman little inconvenience besides the slight leucorrheal discharge which stains her clothing; but often this is indicative of such a change of the lining membrane of the uterus as to render it unfit for the fixation and development of the ovum, even should impregnation take place.

Under normal conditions, during the intermenstrual period, a plug of clear viscid mucus, which is secreted by the glands of the cervical canal, blocks up that passage, but is washed away each month by the menstrual discharge. Under ordinary conditions this obstruction must seriously interfere with the entrance of the spermatozoa into the cavity of the uterus, and renders the former theory, recently revived by Bossi, quite tenable, that impregnation is most likely to occur just after the menstrual epoch.

The vaginal secretion under certain pathologic conditions may become so acid that it induces sterility. Women who suffer m severe vaginal catarrh are frequently sterile, the spermatozoa being found dead in the vagina some hours after copulation, although an examination a shorter time afterward revealed them still alive. In cases where conception takes place in spite of a very acid condition of the vaginal secretion, it is probable that some of the spermatozoa enter the uterus before the secretion has had time to act on them, or possibly the spermatozoa being injected in a mass, the acid secretion is unable to penetrate and kill them all.

The reaction of the normal vaginal mucus is always acid, that of the cervix alkaline; but as the result of the inflammatory condition, the reaction of each is often intensified, especially that of the vagina, which has an exceedingly sour and penetrating odor. This acid discharge, bathing the neck of the uterus, penetrates more or less into the cervical plug and causes coagulation of the alkaline mucus.

The chief constituent of the semen is albumin; agents which affect albuminous substances influence the functional activity of the spermatozoa— heat, concentrated acids, and probably concentrated alkalies. In normal conditions the alkalinity of the seminal fiuid seems to be sufficient to neutralize the acidity of the vaginal secretions, so that the spermatozoa may remain seventeen days or more (Bossi) within the vaginal canal, even during a menstrual period, without having their vitality destroyed.

When hyperacidity of the vaginal secretion is present, it is probable that the fertilizing element is at once rendered inert; but should some of the spermatozoa succeed in reaching the interior of the cervical canal, the increased alkalinity of the secretion there would in all probability put an end to all further progress.

The conditions, then, which appear to prevent fecundation are: First, the absence of the proper nidus for the ovum; second, the obstruction of the cervical canal by a mucus plug; third, increased alkalinity of the cervical secretion, often accompanied by the increased acidity of the vaginal secretion. Three conditions must, then, be determined: First, are there spermatozoa in the semen? Second, do they get into the uterocervical canal? Third, do the secretions in the canal poison the spermatozoa?

"For those who are very anxious for offspring," wrote Marion Sims, "I usually order sexual intercourse on the third, fifth, and seventh days after the flow has ceased; and on the fifth and third days before its return. For the most obvious reasons this would always be before going to bed at night, instead of just before rising in the morning. The horizontal position favors the retention of semen; the erect its expulsion. I am satisfied that too frequent sexual indulgence is fraught with mischief to both parties. It weakens the semen; in other words, that this is not so rich in spermatozoa after too frequent indulgence; and when carried to the extent of a debauch, the fiuid ejaculated may be wholly destitute of spermatozoa. Thus it will be seen that it will be much better to husband the resources of both man and wife."

The Prevention of Conception and the Limitation of Offspring.— Some of the contraindications to procreation are when either parent suffers from a disease which is transmissible, and such diseases frequently manifest themselves only after marriage; when the pregnancy would endanger the mother's life, or even where the pregnancy is a nine months' torture to her; where either parent is suffering from ill health; or where for economical reasons no more children are desired.

If there exists no condition in either parent or in their circumstances why they should not have children, the next consideration due to their children, is how the same may be procreated under the most favorable conditions possible; this condition can only be secured by making the circumtsances such that the mother shall be able to choose the time for their conception when both parents are in the best physical condition. That children should be brought into the world haphazard, as the result of accident, is to degrade the human race below that of the lower animals, where the female admits the male only at the time of the rut, which in the majority of cases occurs only once a year.

Another requisite to bearing healthy children is that the pregnancies shall not follow each other too rapidly. Aside from the consideration for the health of the mother herself, she must be in good physical condition to bear the healthiest children she is capable of giving birth to; and for this there must be from two and a half to three years between the successive pregnancies. The results of overproduction on the children are frequently, that they are sickly, short-lived, or suffer from rickets, cerebral paralysis, idiocy, or imbecility.

And last, but certainly not least, many women become chronic invalids, or are hastened to premature graves, by having children as fast as they possibly can.

The most natural and moral way for the artificial prevention of conception, when on account of ill health or for economic reasons no more children are desired, is to abstain from sexual intercourse. But in the majority of cases the husband will not agree to this, and so the greatest number of methods have come to be used to prevent conception.

Perhaps the most frequent method use to prevent conception is withdrawal before the ejaculation of semen. While this is most injurious to the husband— debility, nervous prostration, and even paralysis are said to ensue— the health of the wife also suffers. If, this interrupted sexual congress is continued for years, there develop gradual nervous disturbances on both sides, and a serious disease of the uterus makes itself felt. The generative organs become engorged with blood, but are not permitted to enjoy relaxation consequent upon the full completion of the act. This engorgement may lead to undue local nutrition, and diffuse growth and proliferation of the connective tissue may take place. Hence the uterine walls become dense and thickened and the nerves compressed. Of course, pain and tenderness and a sense of bearing down will be the result. Flexions and versions may be consequent upon the engorgement. The nerves become shattered, and the woman will be fortunate if she contracts no serious womb trouble.

"It is strange," says John Stuart Mill, "that intemperance in drink or any other appetite, should be condemned so readily, but that incontinence in this respect should always meet not only with indulgence, but with praise. Little improvement can be expected in morality until the producing of too large families is regarded with the same feeling as drunkenness, or any other physical excess."

Sismondi writes: "When our true duties toward those whom we give life are not obscured in the name of a sacred authority, no man will have more children than he can properly bring up. If a woman has a right to decide any question it is how many children she should bear. Whenever it becomes unwise that the family should be increased, justice and humanity require that the husband should impose on himself the same restraint which is submitted to by the unmarried."

In the opinion of Dr. Edward Reich, it is very much to be wished that the function of conception should be placed under the domain of the will. But the strongest appeal has been made for the sake of morality itself; namely, to prevent the crime of abortion. Dr. Raciborski, of Paris, took the position that the prevention of offspring to a certain extent is not only legitimate, but it is to be recommended as a means of public good.

Continence, self-control, and a willingness to deny himself— that is what is required of the husband. But suffering women assure us that this will not suffice; that men refuse to restrain themselves; that it leads to loss of domestic happiness, to illegitimate amours; or that it is injurious physically and mentally; that, in short, such advice is useless because it is impracticable.

Dr. Napheys writes: "Is it amiss to hope that science will find resources, simple and certain, which will enable a woman to let reason and sound judgment, not blind passions, control the increase of her family?"

The Crime of Abortion.— From the moment of conception a new life begins, a new individual exists; another child is added to the family. The mother who deliberately sets about to destroy this life by want of care, or by taking drugs, or by the use of instruments, commits a great crime, and is just as guilty as if she strangled her new-born infant. The crime she commits is child-murder. Women in their frenzy at finding themselves in this condition, and with no slightest idea of the sin that they are committing, are constantly guilty of committing abortions on themselves, or going to professional abortionists to have this crime of child-murder committed. This is another of the sins due to the ignorance of the sex in all matters pertaining to reproduction; and it is a fearfully prevalent one.

Infidelity in Women.— "We have now reached the last infernal circle of the divine comedy of marriage; we are at the depths of the inferno. There is something, I do not know what, terrible in the situation in which a married woman finds herself when an illegitimate love has ruined her for the duties of a wife and mother. As has been so well and strongly expressed by Diderot, infidelity in woman is like incredulity in a priest; it is the last step in human forfeitures; it is for her the great social crime, for it implies all the others.

"Weigh the sufferings of the future, the agonies of years by the ecstasy of half an hour. If this conservative sentiment of the creature, the fear of death, does not stop her, what could be expected of laws? Oh, sublime infamy!"— (Balzac).

PART III.— MATERNITY.

CHAPTER X.

PREGNANCY.

Nature of Conception; Pregnancy Defined; Duration of Pregnancy; the Signs of Pregnancy; Quickening; the Determination of Sex at Will; the Influence of the Male Sexual Element on the Female Organism; Heredity; Hygiene of Pregnancy; Causes of Miscarriage.

> "Happy he
> With such a mother, faith in womankind
> Beats with his bood, and trust in all things high
> Comes easy to him, and though he trip and fall,
> He shall not bind his soul with clay."
>
> — TENNYSON.

Nature of Conception.— Conception, or impregnation, is the union of the germ and the sperm cell, the result of which is a new being. On coition, the semen being received into the female organs, which are at that time in a state of turgescence, the spermatozoa, by means of their own vibratile activity, find their way into the Fallopian tubes, and here come in contact with the ovule.

The ovule is a minute cell with a transparent membrane, within which is the yolk containing the germinal vesicle. The spermatozoon penetrates into the ovule and becomes fused with it. The processes of development begin at once to occur. There is congestion of the uterine mucous membrane out of proportion to the rest of the uterus; the ovum finds lodging here, and becomes surrounded by a membrane which incloses it in a separate sac.

Pregnancy Defined.— Pregnancy begins with conception and ends with parturition; it provides for the nutrition and the expulsion of the embryo and for its nutrition for a short time after birth.

The average duration of pregnancy is ten lunar months, or two hundred and eighty days. The date of the confinement is calculated by reckoning from the date of the last menstrual flow; count backward three months from the date of the first appearance of the last menses; to this add twelve months and seven days, five days being for the average menstrual duration and two days for the possibility of fecundation.

Duration of Pregnancy.— Many difficulties are experienced in determining the date of the expected confinement. As most pregnancies occur in married women, we cannot base any calculations on a single act of coitus. And even if there was but one, all physiologists agree that there is a variable period in different women, and in the same woman at different times, between insemination and the fertilization of the ovum. It is the moment of fecundation, or the union of the germ and sperm cells, which marks the beginning of pregnancy. The uncertainty becomes still greater owing to our inadequate knowledge as to the length of time during which the sexual elements, the ova and the spermatozoa, retain their vitality after liberation from their respective sources. While it is not certainly known, it is probable that the ovum is capable of impregnation any time during its sojourn within the oviduct and before reaching the uterus, or probably for a period of about one week from the time of its escape from the Graafian follicle. The remarkable vitality of the spermatozoa even under less favorable circumstances— direct observation shows that these elements retain their movements for over nine days outside of the body— renders it almost certain that their powers of fertilization are maintained for a long time after they are deposited within the healthy female genital tract; it is believed that the spermatozoa are capable of fertilization after a sojourn of three or more weeks within the oviduct.

Consideration of these facts renders apparent the impossibility of fixing with certainty the date of the beginning of pregnancy, since conception may result from the union of the ovum liberated at the beginning of the period with the spermatozoon introduced at the end of that time; or it may result from the meeting of the male elements already within the oviduct with an ovum discharged a day or two before the occurrence of the menstrual period.

The Signs of Pregnancy.— The cessation of the menstrual period is the sign of the greatest value in women who have been regular; but it must always be remembered that there may be an irregularity of menstruation for the first few months after marriage. The appetite is capricious; morning sickness or nausea in the morning on first getting up is a very common symptom in the early months of pregnancy; enlargement of the abdomen; in the first two months of pregnancy the abdomen is flattened and the umbilicus is depressed; after this the abdomen begins to enlarge. There is also an increase in the size of the breasts, with a deepened color of their areolae and later a watery secretion. The external genitals become swollen and of a bluish color. Feeling of the fetal movements— that is, the movements of the small parts of the child in the womb— by the mother is not always reliable, since gas in the intestines has sometimes been mistaken for this. These signs are more valuable when several exist together.

The nausea and vomiting of pregnancy, the so-called morning sickness, consists of nausea accompanied often by vomiting or retching of a glairy fiuid, showing itself most frequently on rising in the morning, but sometimes appearing after breakfast. It is aggravated by the assumption of the erect position. It may begin within a few days, but as a rule it does not show itself until the fourth week of pregnancy; and it generally ceases about the fourth month, rarely persisting throughout the entire time. In the majority of cases it does not sensibly impair the health. It is a sympathetic disorder reflected from the uterus; it is aggravated by indigestible food, by sexual excitement, and by emotional disturbances; it is most marked in first pregnancies and in women of highly emotional natures. It is not infrequently due to some inflammation of the uterus or erosion about the external orifice, and disappears on the removal of the cause.

Mammary Changes. — During pregnancy the mammary glands are in immediate sympathy with the growing reproductive organs of the pelvis; consequently a genuine physiologic enlargement commences in these organs from the beginning of gestation. Their glandular structure becomes larger, fuller, and firmer; a sensation of weight or pricking is felt by the patient; the veins become more prominent. The nipples also become enlarged, more elongated, and somewhat erect. Surrounding the nipple is the areola; this becomes darker in color.

In most women a drop of watery fiuid, the so-called colostrum, may be squeezed out from the nipple at the end of the third month of pregnancy.

The signs of pregnancy are divided into the presumptive, the probable, and the positive. The presumptive signs are: menstrual suppression, morning sickness, irritable bladder, mental and emotional phenomena. The probable signs are: mammary changes, abdominal enlargement, changes in the neck of the womb, and certain changes which are felt on bimanual examination. The positive signs are: feeling the various parts of the fetus, active movements of the fetus, and hearing the fetal heart sounds.

Functional disturbances of the bladder are quite often noticeable in the early part of the pregnancy. In the first part of the pregnancy the bladder is dragged upon, and later it is pressed upon by the enlarged uterus so that the bladder capacity is lessened and frequency of urination is the result. In the fourth month, when the uterus ascends into the abdominal cavity, these bladder symptoms subside, until the very close of the pregnancy, when by the descent of the now greatly enlarged uterus there may be even incontinence of urine.

Changes in the Abdomen. – During the first two months of the pregnancy there is a flattening of the abdominal surface, due to the descent of the uterus into the pelvic cavity, thus slightly dragging the bladder downward and drawing the umbilicus inward. In the latter part of the fourth month there is noticeable a slight abdominal enlargement, and the umbilicus is no longer sunken. By the end of the fourth month the base of the uterus has risen two inches above the symphysis, and at the end of the thirty-eighth week it touches the lower extremity of the breast-bone; the umbilicus has been for many weeks protruding; during the last two weeks of pregnancy the uterus again descends and the woman feels more comfortable.

On the inspection of the abdomen of a pregnant woman there will be noticed a brown line which extends from the umbilicus to the pubes, and all over the surface the presence of striae, or long purple grooves, due to the distention of the abdomen; on the sides of the abdomen and down the thighs, red, blue, or white markings, like cicatrices, may be seen.

Quickening.— Quickening is the sensation experienced by the mother as the result of the active fetal movements of the child in the womb. These movements are first felt between the eighteenth and the twentieth week; the common rule is that quickening occurs at the middle of pregnancy; that is, at four and a half months. As pregnancy advances these active motions increase in frequency and become more marked. When felt or seen by the physician, as can be done in the sixth month, fetal movements constitute a positive sign of pregnancy.

The Determination of Sex at Will.— Although this has always been a question of great interest, and the subject of much experimentation, no rule can as yet be given by which the parents can know in advance of the birth of the child what the sex will be. Dr. Schenck's theory is that the ruling factor in determining the sex is the food partaken of by the mother.

Furst believes that the differentiation may occur before, during, and a little while after the impregnation; that the chances of the development of one or another sex in one and the same woman may vary before final differentiation occurs. It is impossible to determine the sex of the embryo before the tenth week of fetal life. The cause of the differentiation, he believes, lies largely in the good or bad state of the health of the parents; in the first instance there being an excess of females, and in the latter an excess of males, relatively speaking. He believes that there is an excess of male children when conception takes place during the post-menstrual anemia. He has investigated one hundred and ninety-three cases carefully in regard to the probable date of conception after menstruation, and there is a notable increase of male births over female in the cases where conception occurred in the first five days after menstruation; that is to say, where the woman is not so well nourished as later.

Dr. J. Griffith Davis gives as the result of her experiments in this direction, that when conception takes place three days before the menstrual period or within forty-eight hours afterward, the child will be a girl; when conception takes place ten days after the period, the child will be a boy.

Although there are a greater number of the female than the male sex in all parts of the world where reliable statistics have been taken, in all civilized countries the proportion of male births is greater than that of females. There is a greater tendency of the male offspring to die earlier, and this is seen even before birth, in the proportion of three to two. For this reason the stronger sex as applied to men has been regarded by some authors as a misnomer. They are physically weaker in early life and succumb more readily to noxious influences.

The relative age of the parents is said to be another factor in determining the sex of the children. Seniority on the father's side gives an excess of male children; equality in the age of the parents gives a slight preponderance of females; seniority on the mother's side gives an excess of females. Men, and especially scholars, who pass a sedentary life and who exhaust their nervous force to a great extent, beget more girls than boys; so, also, a very advanced age on the part of the man diminishes the number of male offspring.

The Influence of the Male Sexual Element on the Female Organism.— Dr. Alexander Harvey, of Aberdeen, has adopted the theory of fetal inoculation. He believes that the effect is first due to the influence of the male element upon the ovum, which, in consequence of the subsequent close attachment and freely intercommunicating blood-vessels between the modified embryo and the mother, inoculates the condition of the mother with the qualities of the male; and so, on the subsequent impregnation by another male, the offspring resembles the first male and not its real parent. He even goes further, and says that it is conceivable, by successive impregnations effected by him, that the influence may be increased, and if so the younger children begotten by him, rather than the elder, might be expected, *ceteris paribus,* to bear their father's image. And as regards the mother, he suggests the question, whether there is not something in the popular notion that in the course of years the wife comes to resemble the husband; and that not merely in respect of temper, disposition, or habits of thought, but in bodily appearance, which may be referable to this influence exerted by the husband on her constitution, through the medium of the fetuses *in utero*.

> "Yet it shall be; thou shalt lower to his level day by day,
> What is fine within thee growing coarse to sympathize with clay.
> As the husband is the wife is; thou art mated with a clown,
> And the grossness of his nature will have weight to drag thee down.
> He will hold thee, when his passion shall have spent its novel force,
> Something better than his dog, a little dearer than his horse."

Darwin, on the other hand, considers it a most improbable hypothesis that the mere blood of one individual should affect the reproductive organs of another individual in such a manner as to affect the subsequent offspring. The analogy, he says, from the direct action of the foreign pollen on the ovaries and seed coats of the mother plant strongly supports the belief that the male element acts directly on the reproductive organs of the female, and not through the intervention of the crossed embryo.

Dr. John Brown, in reviewing the subject, says it must be conceded that the male element has an influence on the female, over and above its fertilizing influence upon the ovum. The limit of this influence is at present unknown.

Heredity.— Girls are more apt to resemble their fathers in mental traits, disposition, and constitution; while boys take after their mothers. Boys procreated by intelligent mothers will be intelligent; while it does not always follow that the sons of intelligent fathers are intelligent. The poets Burns, Ben Johnson, Goethe, Walter Scott, Byron, and Lamartine were all born of women remarkable for vivacity and brilliance of language.

Hygiene of Pregnancy. — The health and perfection of the child depend largely upon the health and perfection of the parents at the time of its conception, as well as upon the condition of the mother during the pregnancy. Even when both parents possess a strong constitution, but one or both of them is suffering from a temporary exhaustion or malaise, the child will be born below the standard of health it ought to possess. Children born during the first year of married life seldom equal in health the children born of the same parents later; they are not only apt to be sickly, but the liability to premature death is greatly increased. For this reason it is better that the first year of married life should be allowed to pass without conception taking place. A child begotten in an intoxicated or depraved condition of a parent may be depraved itself in the same way, and is apt to be feeble-minded or idiotic.

It must be borne in mind that prenatal culture of some sort begins at the time of conception; and that on the mental as well as on the physical state of the mother, the health as well as the disposition of the child will depend to no slight extent. The prospective mother who constantly gives way to her feelings does a wrong to her unborn child. The mother is at this time more impressionable, more nervous, and more irritable than is natural to her; and while her family should make a certain allowance for her condition, she, on her part, should not allow herself to give way to her morbid feelings. The prospective mother should not lead a life of self-indulgence, on the one hand, or, on the other, should not be weighed down with cares; she should interest herself in her usual duties, and be relieved of all anxiety possible.

Dress. — The clothing must be loose, and all compression about the waist and abdomen must be especially avoided. If the woman wears corsets, she must take them off at once, and substitute a Ferris or some similar hygienic waist. The corset prevents the proper development of the abdominal muscles, which play so important a role in the expulsion of the child from the womb, as well as in the proper growth and development of the fetus itself. If the woman has already borne children, and toward the end of the pregnancy the abdomen becomes pendulous, she will very materially add to her comfort by swearing a muslin abdominal bandage.

A woolen undersuit, or undervest and drawers, with high neck and long sleeves, must be worn winter and summer; the grade of the wool to be adapted to the season of the year. The especial necessity for wearing wool next the skin during the pregnancy is because of the intimate relation between the skin and the kidneys. Any chilling of the body at this time is apt to lead to the congestion of the kidneys. If there is already any congestion of the kidneys present, or any abdominal pain, in addition to the undersuit an abdominal bandage should be worn. These bandages come woven in ribbed woolen, and fit the body snugly. This bandage is to be constantly worn, and, of course, changed at night. During the cold weather the stockings should also be of wool. Under no circumstances are garters allowed to be worn, as they form a constriction around the leg and interfere with the return of the venous blood to the heart, and so increase the tendency to the formation of the varicose veins. It is better not to use any means to hold the stockings up; they will be kept sufficiently well in place by the under-drawers. Low shoes should never be worn except in the hottest weather. It is of the greatest importance that the woman should be impressed with the necessity of the avoidance of taking cold, since any lung or kidney trouble is a serious complication of pregnancy.

Diet. – The diet is the same as that at any other time, only it is more necessary to guard against anything which is likely to cause indigestion. In other words, the diet should be plain, simple, and easy of digestion; nutritious and partaken of at regular intervals. In the latter part of pregnancy owing to the pressure of the enlarged uterus on the stomach, the food may have to be partaken of in smaller quantities and at shorter intervals. At this time also the appetite is abnormally large. Where it does not disagree with the patient, milk is the best adjuvant possible to the diet.

Constipation. – Constipation is the rule of pregnancy. This is due to the great pressure that the enlarged uterus makes on the bowel; and as important as it is at all times to keep the bowels regular, it is at this time more necessary than ever that the woman should have the bowels well evacuated every day. A retention of fecal matter in the body causes the reabsorption into the blood of the toxic matters, with the resulting headaches, dizziness, loss of appetite, and intense nervousness. To obviate this tendency to constipation, plenty of fruit and vegetables should be eaten, as well as cereals if the woman is taking a good deal of outdoor exercise, otherwise the latter had better be omitted. The woman should drink plenty of water — at least three pints a day; this acts as a laxative as well as to flush out the kidneys. If, in spite of all these measures, constipation still persists, as it probably will, a seidlitz powder can be taken the first thing on rising in the morning; or from one teaspoonful to one tablespoonful of the effervescing granules of the phosphate of soda in a glass of water, also to be taken on rising in the morning; or one-half grain of the solid extract of cascara sagrada night and morning. The object of these is to keep the bowels open, but purgation must always be avoided.

Bladder Symptoms. — If there is any irritability of the bladder, any scalding on urination, or a very great frequency of emptying the bladder in the early months of pregnancy, a physician should be consulted at once; in the last months of pregnancy there is a desire to evacuate the bladder frequently, and sometimes at the last there is an incontinence of urine, which is due to the descent of the uterus and the great pressure on the bladder; this condition disappears with the confinement.

Leucorrhea. — If this is present to any marked degree, the vaginal douche should be continued throughout the pregnancy; the temperature of the douche should be from 110° to 112° F.; it must never be taken very hot or very cold. The fountain syringe should be used, and the bag should not be hung more than three feet above the bed, so that there shall not be too much force to the stream of water.

Baths. — Warm tub-baths may be taken throughout the pregnancy, but never oftener than twice a week, and the woman should never stay in the tub longer than is absolutely necessary for the bath, as otherwise the bath is too enervating. A daily sponge-bath of cool or cold salt water at a temperature of from 80° to 70° F., and in the proportion of a pint of rock or sea salt to a gallon of water is most invigorating, and counteracts many of the nervous symptoms and promotes sleep and good digestion. The temperature of the room in which this bath is taken should be 72° F. Shower-baths cause too great a shock to the nervous system, and they as well as foot-baths must be prohibited. Sitz-baths at a temperature from 110°

to 90° F. may be taken just before retiring throughout the pregnancy. The frequency and duration of the bath as well as the temperature should be regulated by the attending physician. In cases of intense nervousness and insomnia these baths have an excellent sedative effect. A pregnant woman must never under any circumstances take ocean baths, since there is always great danger that the shock of the waves will cause an abortion. Sea-voyages should be avoided because of the severe nausea and vomiting, as well as the danger that the lurching of the vessel may cause miscarriage.

The sewing-machine is a tabooed thing for the pregnant woman, because of the jarring of the pelvis which it produces. Sweeping of heavy carpets is also injurious. There must be no lifting of heavy pieces of furniture, and especially no lifting from the floor, as it interferes with the circulation in the uterus and is apt to produce miscarriage.

Driving in an easy carriage over smooth roads is permissible; dogcarts, or any conveyance which produces much jolting, must be avoided; and while driving is good, the woman should not do her own driving, on account of the danger of the jars that would be caused by the sudden pulling of the horse upon the lines. Horseback-riding and bicycling are, of course, forbidden, as are also golf, tennis, and dancing.

Exercise. – Exercise in the open air should be taken every day, when the weather is suitable, and walking is the best form of exercise. The amount will be regulated to some extent by what the woman has been accustomed to taking, and it should always stop short of fatigue. The woman should live as much as possible in the open air, and she should attend to her ordinary duties about the house. Long railway journeys are always objectionable.

Hemorrhoids or piles are very often troublesome toward the close of the pregnancy. To overcome this, the patient should lie down immediately after the bowel movement, and remain in the recumbent position for ten or fifteen minutes. In addition, care should be taken to secure a loose movement of the bowels. Should the piles come down, applications of cloths wrung out of hot water, and held well pressed against the bowel, should be made; the piles should then be pressed back until the finger feels that the mass has been pushed above the second constriction of the bowel, which is felt to exist at about two inches above the sphincter ani muscle. Should these means not suffice, the physician must be consulted at once.

Swelling and pain of the external genitals and of the lower limbs are best relieved by the recumbent position. Should the veins of the legs be much enlarged or the feet swollen, the patient should have compression made by the wearing of elastic stockings. Or in some cases a bandage is sufficient; in this case the bandage may be made of muslin; it should be three inches wide, and, beginning at the toes, should extend up as high as the enlargement of the veins continues. This bandage should be freshly applied every morning before rising.

Pain caused by the stretching of the skin may be relieved by the inunction of the skin with cottonseed or cocoanut oil. For severe pain in the small of the back, rubbing with soap liniment or alcohol will be found useful.

Mental Occupation. — Important as this always is, it is doubly so now. The mind should be constantly and pleasantly occupied, but no severe study should be indulged in. The emotional susceptibility is generally somewhat increased. The pregnant woman, quite excitable and irritable, readily responds to influences by which in the non-gravid condition she could not be affected. Sometimes she feels unusually well, is intellectually brightened and more active, and says she is positively happier. At other times she is despondent and morose.

Physiologists admit and observation proves that maternal emotions do affect the development and the exterior of the fetus; likewise the mental organization of the fetus may be affected. All unpleasant news, frights, and physical shocks, also scenes of suffering and distress, must be avoided, as the mind is particularly impressionable at this time. Around the patient should be thrown a gentle and protective care, and she should be treated with the considerate kindness which her condition demands. Theatres and all places where there will be a large assemblage of people should be avoided, as the close air and general bad ventilation are apt to produce vertigo and sometimes attacks of fainting.

Sleep. — During pregnancy a large amount of sleep is required; there should be eight hours spent in sleep at night, and one hour every afternoon. Pregnant women should never do any night watching. There is unusual necessity for good ventilation during sleep at this time.

The Marital Relation. — Coitus is, as a rule, distasteful to pregnant women. It is for the best interest of the wife as well as for that of the child that all marital relation should be suspended at this time. Even uncivilized nations have condemned the privilege of sexual intercourse during pregnancy, and have visited punishment on the offender. If these relations are not wholly suspended, they must at least be at those periods which correspond to the time at which the woman would have been unwell had she not been pregnant. To the continuance of these relations throughout the pregnancy is due much of the suffering of the wife, not only then, but at the time of the labor as well; and the nourishment of the child is interfered with.

Causes of Miscarriage. — Hemorrhoids; straining at stool; excessive intercourse in the newly married; nursing; ocean-bathing; overexertion; overexcitement; a fall; any violent emotion; anger; sudden or excessive joy; a fright; running; dancing; horseback-riding; riding in a heavily built carriage over rough roads; great fatigue; lifting heavy weights; the abuse of purgative medicines; disease or displacements of the womb; and a general condition of ill health.

The danger of miscarriage is greatest during the first three months of pregnancy. Miscarriage is a fruitful source of disease and often of danger to wives; it is said that thirty-seven out of every hundred pregnant women miscarry. Miscarriage is most apt to occur during the first pregnancy; and great care should be taken to prevent this, as the habit is easily established, and after one miscarriage has occurred, another is likely to follow, so that it is sometimes with the greatest difficulty that the woman can be made to carry the fetus to full term. Artificially produced abortions are not an infrequent cause of sterility; the young wife becomes pregnant, and has an abortion produced because she is not yet ready to give up all her pleasures; and eventually when she does become very anxious to have a child such an extent of uterine disease has been produced by the abortions that she cannot conceive.

To Prevent Miscarriage. — The life must be free from all excitement, and must be as quiet as possible without becoming monotonous; especial care must be exercised at the return of the dates for the menstrual periods.

The symptoms of miscarriage are a show of blood, more or less profuse, with intense abdominal pain; on the slightest show of blood the patient should go to bed at once and the physician should be sent for.

CHAPTER XI.

THE CONFINEMENT.

Preparation for the Confinement; Signs of Approaching Labor; Symptoms of Actual Labor; the Confinement-bed; the Process of Labor.

> "To my conception one generation of educated mothers would do more for the regeneration of the race than all other human agencies combined; and it is an instruction of the head they need, and not of the heart. The doctrine of responsibility has been ground into Christian mothers above what they are able to bear."
>
> — ISABELLE BEECHER HOOKER.

Preparations for the Confinement. — The right time to engage the physician who is to take charge of the woman at her confinement is just so soon as the woman knows that she is pregnant. It used to be argued that, since giving birth to children was a physiologic process, there was no necessity for the woman to consult the physician until he was sent for when the labor pains began. Take the case of the woman who is for the first time pregnant; she is absolutely at sea; she has not the least idea how she ought to feel, what she ought to do or to leave undone; the result is that she often has a miscarriage which is the source of the greatest disappointment to her husband and herself, or she suffers very unnecessarily throughout the entire pregnancy, has a difficult labor, and perhaps gives birth to a sickly child.

The educated physician will explain to her what symptoms are normal and what are pathologic, and often he will be able to entirely cure the latter. It is now a well-established fact that the most serious complications of the pregnancy, and of the labor itself are caused by severe congestion or disease of the kidneys. The condition of the kidneys can only be determined by frequent examinations of the urine; during the early months of pregnancy these examinations are made once a month, and during the last month they are made every week. The amount of urine passed in the normal condition is three pints a day.

Nowhere, perhaps, is the constant vigilance of the physician so well rewarded as in the careful oversight of the pregnant woman. She goes through her entire pregnancy feeling well, and often the greatest discomfort that she suffers is due to her size; her labor and her lying-in are normal, and she gives birth to a healthy child.

Engagement of the Nurse. – This is generally left to the physician in charge of the case, since he is responsible for the safe delivery of the woman; but if the patient has any decided choice in the matter, it is acceded to unless there should be some very valid objections, and the physician always sends the nurse in view for that case to see the patient in order to ascertain if she is personally agreeable to the patient.

Choice of Room for the Confinement and Lying-in. – The room should be light, sunny, and well ventilated; it should not be too near a water-closet. In the city as quiet a room as possible should be selected, and one that is well removed from the rest of the house, so that if necessary perfect quiet can be maintained. The room should be as cheery as possible.

The dress of the mother during the lying-in consists of a merino undervest, with high neck and long sleeves, and a nightgown, which shall be open all the way down the front. The gowns should be made of light muslin or of cambric; and there should be a sufficient number so that they may be changed every day.

Six abdominal bandages should be provided. These are made of light muslin, and they should be eighteen inches wide and long enough to go once and a third around the patient's hips at the sixth month of pregnancy, or about one yard and a quarter long; they may be made straight or to fit the patient at the sixth month. This bandage is fastened down the front; it is applied directly after the labor, and adds greatly to the patient's comfort during the lying-in.

The vulvar pads used during the lying-in are the antiseptic absorbent pads which can be obtained at any place where surgical dressings are sold; they are made of absorbent cotton, covered with cheesecloth, and sterilized.

There must be a sufficiently generous supply of sheets so that they can be changed every day, and the drawsheet as often as may be required. Nothing is so important to a good lying-in as to have a clean, well-ventilated room, and plenty of fresh bed-linen. Cleanliness is the first requisite to antisepsis, and this is the secret of avoiding puerperal fever.

Articles to be provided for the confinement are:

1. An oblong douche-pan of agate-ware.
2. An agate bed-pan.
3. A bath thermometer.
4. Two pieces of rubber sheeting; one, one yard square, and the other two yards square.
5. Two sterilized bed-pads, 30 inches square by 3 to 4 inches thick.
6. Three dozen antiseptic absorbent pads.
7. One pound of sterilized absorbent cotton; twelve yards of cheese-cloth.
8. Six abdominal bandages, eighteen inches wide, preferably made to fit the figure at the sixth month of gestation.
9. Two hand-scrubs.
10. Four ounces of the tincture of green soap.
11. Bottle of corrosive sublimate tablets.
12. Four ounces of powdered boric acid.
13. Half a pint of good whisky.
14. Two ounces of aromatic spirits of ammonia.

15. Two ounces of aqua ammonia.
16. One pint of alcohol.
17. Two tubes sterilized white vaselin.
18. Plenty of large and small safety-pins.
19. Hot-water bag.
20. New fountain syringe, to hold four quarts; with glass nozzle.
21. One small basin for vomited matter.
22. Two very large agate basins or wash-bowls for washing doctor's hands and for antiseptic solutions.
23. Vessel for after-birth.
24. Three large pitchers; one for boiling water, one for cold boiled water, and one for antiseptic solution.
25. Tumbler for boric acid solution for washing baby's eyes, with fine old linen sterilized.
26. One dozen freshly laundered sheets, and two dozen towels.
27. Stocking-drawers, muslin.
28. Change of night-clothing warmed for the mother.
29. A warm blanket to receive the baby.
30. An infant bath-tub.
31. A large piece of oil-cloth to protect the floor.*

* Van Horn & Co., Park Avenue and 41st Street, New York, keep an obstetric outfit, containing many of the above articles, cleansed, sterilized, and packed in a box ready for use, so that they remain intact until needed. The price of this outfit is $16.50.

Baby's Outfit. — Four flannel bandages, to be made of fine, soft flannel, four inches wide, to go once and a third around the body. The edges may be pinked or whipped, but should never be hemmed; a tape is sewed on double, the ends passing around the body, and so the bandage is fastened without pinning.

Six merino shirts, with high neck and long sleeves, made to button down the front.

Cotton diaper napkins, not too large; old soft ones are preferable.

Long merino stockings which can be pinned to the napkin.

Flannel petticoats, not too long; these may be made on muslin bands, which are held up on the shoulders by means of straps. The essential in all the clothing is that it should be sufficiently loose.

Dress-slips should not be so elaborate that they cannot be washed and changed with sufficient frequency; and not so long that the baby's feet will be hampered in their movements by them. All of baby's clothes but the dress should be fastened by safety-pins.

Baby's basket should contain:

1. One outfit of clothes.
2. One tube of sterilized tape.
3. A pair of blunt-pointed scissors.
4. Large and small safety-pins.
5. Pieces of fine old linen; old handkerchiefs are the best.
6. A soft hair-brush.
7. A powder box and puff, with talcum powder.
8. Two tubes of sterilized white vaselin.
9. Two soft towels.
10. Castile soap.
11. Single-bulb syringe; so-called "eye and ear syringe."
12. A woolen shawl or wrap.

If there is no nurse available before the labor sets in, and it is necessary for the patient to see to the sterilizing of the above articles, she should first scrub off all pitchers, basins, and other utensils, as well as the douche-pan, fountain syringe, and rubber sheeting, with a brush and hot soap-suds; the hand-scrubs are to be well washed; then each article should be pinned separately in coarse towels, and put to boil for half an hour in an ordinary wash-boiler. The articles so boiled are then dried without removing the towels, put away, and not opened till the time of the labor.

The abdominal bandages must be laundried and pinned up in separate towels until they are needed. The cheese-cloth must be laundried and then sterilized.

The vulvar pads should be pinned in an old napkin, in packages of half a dozen each; and one package is sterilized at a time by placing it in the oven until the outer covering is scorched. The linen for the baby's eyes and the cheese-cloth are treated in the same way; they are to be cut up into small pieces and sterilized as needed.

Signs of Approaching Labor.— About two weeks before labor there is a sinking of the womb. At the beginning of the ninth lunar month this was at the end of the breast-bone; it now descends to a point midway between this and the navel; the abdomen becomes smaller, the pressure on the lungs is relieved, and the woman breathes more freely. But at the same time that the woman is relieved of the pressure on the chest, she experiences increase of the troubles in the lower extremities. There is an increase of the bladder symptoms, with a desire for frequent unrination. Constipation becomes more troublesome, and there may be hemorrhoids; the veins of the lower extremities may become greatly enlarged.

There is an increased fullness of the external genitals and a greatly augmented amount of mucous discharge. There is a feeling of anxiety and nervousness, with depression of spirits.

During the last two weeks of pregnancy patients are apt to have cramp-like pains in the lower part of the abdomen. These are often mistaken for labor pains. True labor pains are characterized by starting in the back, extending around the abdomen and toward the pubes and down the thighs; they come at more or less regular intervals of half to three-quarters of an hour, and increase in intensity with a decrease in the intervals. A strong pain is apt to be followed by two weaker ones. The so-called false pains are irregular in their occurrence.

Symptoms of Actual Labor.— First is generally the show; this is a discharge of mucous tinged with blood; at the same time the true labor pains set in. When the patient or nurse is in any doubt as to the character of the pains, or when the show appears, the physician should be summoned at once. Other symptoms are frequent desire to empty the bladder and bowels, and a sensation of shivering.

The Confinement-Bed.— A single bed is much more convenient, but it is rarely found in a private house. The double bed is arranged as follows: The hair mattress is covered with a large rubber sheet, which is pinned with safety-pins at the corners and tucked well under the mattress; the rubber sheet must not be drawn too tightly for fear of tearing. Over this comes the sheet, and over the upper half of the bed, the draw-sheet; this is a sheet folded four double, which goes across the bed so as to come under the hips of the patient, and is tucked under the mattress at both sides. The object of this is so that it may be frequently and easily changed without disturbing the patient. The sheet, blanket, and spread which are to serve as a covering after delivery are folded back and placed on the left side of the bed.

The lower right-hand corner of the bed — the right side of the bed is that side which is toward the right hand as one stands facing the foot-board — is arranged for the confinement; on this is fastened the smaller rubber sheet, and over this the sheet is folded, and both are fastened down with safety-pins. The pillow for the patient should be placed at the upper and inner corner of the square. After the delivery the patient is lifted to the upper part of the bed and the temporary dressing is removed. A sheet and blanket are used for a covering during the confinement.

Before the labor begins it is well to fasten up the vest and gown, so that they will not be soiled, as it is important that the patient shall be moved as little as possible after the labor, as all movements tend to increase the bleeding.

The floor oilcloth must be spread at the side of the bed which is made up for the confinement, and should extend slightly under the bed.

A bureau in the room should contain the mother's and baby's clothing, bed-linen, towels, and any other articles which will be needed, all properly arranged.

The clothing for the mother and baby will be placed where it will keep warm, and the infant bathtub will be in readiness in case of sudden need for it.

All water used about the confinement must have been carefully sterilized in advance. The best way to sterilize the water is by boiling it in a large wash-boiler; whatever vessel is used must be scrupulously clean, and ought to be new. The vessel is covered over, and the water is allowed to boil for half an hour; it is then, still covered, set aside to cool. There should be three gallons each of sterilized hot and cold water; since in case of an emergency there must be plenty of water ready for use.

The various articles ordered in the confinement outfit will be at hand ready for use. It is the duty of the nurse to have everything ready for the doctor before his arrival. The patient should have a full warm tub-bath, fresh night-clothes put on, and an enema should be at once given to unload the bowels, and this even though there may have been a bowel movement only a few hours previously. The patient should remain in bed until the arrival of the doctor. After an examination has assured the latter that all is right, she may be allowed to go around the room, with a wrapper thrown on over the night-gown.

Conveniently near the bed should be a small table, covered with one or two freshly laundried towels. This table should have on it a wash-basin, a hand-brush, soap and hot water, an antiseptic solution, scissors, a ligature for the navel, and a suitable aseptic lubricant for the hands.

The Process of Labor.— The process of labor is divided into three stages. The first stage is that of dilatation; by which is meant the stretching of the mouth of the womb so that the child may pass through. At the first confinement this stage lasts about fifteen hours; at subsequent labors the length of this stage is much shorter, the average time being eight hours. The pains during this stage are sharp and cutting, and they are accompanied by a slight show of blood. The patient is fretful and nervous

The second stage of labor is called that of expulsion, because in this stage the uterus contracts down together with the abdominal muscles to expel the child from the womb and the vagina into the world. The duration of this stage in the first confinement is about an hour and a half.

The third stage of labor includes the time from the expulsion of the child till the coming away of the after-birth; the average length of this stage is from twenty minutes to half an hour.

The average length of time for the first labor is seventeen hours; and for subsequent labors from eight to eleven hours.

The bag of waters is the sac of membranes in which the child is inclosed. It contains a liquid in which the child floats; the object of the water is to protect the child from sudden shocks or any kind of injury during pregnancy. During labor this membrane with its contained water serves as a dilating wedge to assist in the opening of the womb, and it also protects the child from the direct contraction of the uterus upon it. When the waters break prematurely, the labor is much longer and more tedious; normally this should not occur before the mouth of the womb is fully dilated.

The pains of the second stage of labor are of a bearing down character, and constantly increase in force and frequency; the climax being reached as the head passes through the vulvar orifice.

A child usually lies in the womb with the head downward; the reason of this is that there is more room in the upper part of the uterus, and as the small parts of the child as it is folded upon itself take up the most space, they occupy this position, while the head lies just above the pubes. The normal position of the child is: the head is flexed on the chest, the legs on the thighs and the thighs on the abdomen, and the hands are folded across the chest. And so the child is usually born head first.

During the stage of expulsion the head of the child is forced down slightly during each pain, to recede a little during the intervals between the pains; in this way the vagina and its external orifice are gradually stretched so that the head of the child may pass through without tearing the parts. If the head is allowed to pass through suddenly, or where the labors are rapid, as in the case of women who have given birth to several children, much mischief may be done by tearing the soft parts.

After the birth of the head there is a short interval of rest, when the shoulders are born; the rest of the body easily slips out; and with the expulsion of the after-birth the labor is over.

At the very beginning of labor the patient should be given a full warm tub-bath, and make an entire change of linen. She will usually prefer to be dressed in her night-clothing, over which during the first stage she may wear a loose wrapper; a sterilized napkin should be worn over the vulva during this stage. During the first stage, as a rule, the patient should not be confined to bed until the dilatation is well advanced; she is generally more comfortable if she is allowed to move around the room, and the pains are thereby advanced.

The only way in which the physician can determine whether labor has begun is by making an internal examination; and this will enable him to decide as to whether it is necessary to remain or not.

The nurse should always wear a wash dress in the confinement and lying-in room.

If the labor is long, nourishment in the form of beef-tea, broths, and milk may be given. No stimulants should be given without the direction of the physician. The frequent taking of cold water is permissible.

At the beginning of the labor the family and friends must be excluded from the room, and it must be kept as quiet and as cheerful as possible.

Toilet of the Patient. — The newly born child is received in a small blanket, is well wrapped, and laid in a warm place. The nurse then turns her attention to the mother; the external genitals and soiled parts of the body are cleansed with sterilized cheese-cloth wrung out of an antiseptic solution; if the body-linen has become soiled, it is also changed, and all blood-stained articles are removed from the bed. The patient is then carefully lifted up on the permanent bed, and the vulvar pad and the abdominal bandage are applied; after which the patient is allowed to rest.

CHAPTER XII.

LYING-IN.

Management of the Lying-in; Lactation; Nursing.

> "'Tis is ourselves that we are thus or thus. Our bodies are our gardens; to the which, our wills are gardeners."— "*Othello.*"

Management of the Lying-in.— Immediately after the delivery the first essential for the patient is absolute quiet and rest; the room must be kept quiet and darkened, and ordinarily the patient is allowed to fall into a light sleep. During the first few hours after labor the best position for the mother is flat on the back, with only a small pillow under the head. After the first twenty-four hours the patient may be allowed to turn on the side as she prefers. Since absolute rest is the first requisite for the patient, she must be left alone with the nurse, who must see that she does not fall into too deep a sleep. If the child's cries disturb the mother, it must be taken into another room.

The lying-in room must be kept free from all odors, all soiled clothing must be at once removed from the room, and good ventilation must be insured, being careful to prevent any drafts.

While the patient is asleep, and after the baby has been attended to, the nurse should place all blood-stained articles in cold water to soak. If in the city, the after-birth may be burned in the furnace or range; it should be well covered with coal. In the country the after-birth can be buried in a deep hole.

During the first two or three days the vulvar dressings should be changed from every three to six hours, and at all times as often as they are soiled. Each time that the dressing is renewed the external genitals and their immediate surroundings are to be carefully cleansed with sterilized water, and finally washed with a solution of boric acid, in the proportion of one tablespoonful of boric acid to one quart of water. It is convenient to keep this solution mixed and on hand, as it takes some little time to prepare it; it should be kept in a strength double that which is desired, so that it may be diluted with warm water to give the desired temperature. This solution may be poured over the parts from a small pitcher, the douche-pan having been placed under the patient before the washing began. After labor the vulva is very sensitive, so that while the greatest care must be used to remove all clots of blood and the discharge, there must be no brisk rubbing of the parts. No blood-stained linen should be permitted to remain about the patient or the bed.

Since the lying-in woman perspires freely, her skin ought to be frequently cleansed by sponging with a weak solution of alcohol in tepid water; this should be followed by friction with a towel until the skin is in a glow. Cleanliness of the bed is promoted by the use of a draw-sheet, which is a sheet folded to four thicknesses and placed beneath the patient's hips in such a way that the upper edge of the sheet shall come under the lower part of the pillows. Air and light must be freely admitted at all times in order that the room may be bright and cheerful. For the first few weeks the eyes of the newborn infant should be shielded from all strong light.

Visitors. — For the first week after the confinement the patient should see no visitors. Even the husband or mother should not remain in the room long at a time. Nothing of a disagreeable nature should be told to the patient; and whoever goes into the sick-room should always carry the most cheerful manner, as it is highly necessary that the patient should be kept mentally as well as physically quiet at this time.

Diet. — For the first twenty-four hours the diet must be restricted to liquids, and in most cases nothing is given until the patient has had a few hours' rest. The first thing that is given to the patient should be a cup of warm milk or tea. Milk is the best diet; this may be varied with beef-tea, bouillon, mutton or chicken broth; any of these broths may be made with rice or barley to vary the flavor, but these must not be given to the patient. The patient should have six ounces of the liquid every two hours during the day and every three hours during the night.

On the second day bread well toasted through may be added to any of the liquids. On the third day stewed or baked apples should be added to the diet. On the fourth day, and from this on, the patient will have regular meals, but the diet must be a plain one. For breakfast, stale bread, a soft-boiled egg, fruit, and a cup of tea, not too strong. For dinner, which should always be given in the middle of the day, an oyster-stew or clam broth, a lamb chop, or a very small piece of beefsteak or chicken; but with these there must be no gravies or dressings; a potato baked in the skin; raw tomatoes, if in season; apple sauce or cranberry; celery; junket, plain corn-starch, lemon jelly, plain cup-custard. From this list the diet must be arranged so as to give as much variety as possible from day to day. Midway between breakfast and dinner, and again in the middle of the afternoon, the patient should have a glass of milk. The diet should be generous, but simple.

Urination. — The feeble condition of the bladder in the first few hours after delivery frequently leads to the retention of urine. Owing to the copious secretion of urine which is so common at this time, painful and injurious distention of the bladder may result. The patient should therefore endeavor to pass her urine in at least six hours after labor, whether she feels any inclination to do so or not; the sound of running water or warm fomentations over the bladder, warm water in the douche-pan, and moderate pressure applied by the hand over the suprapubic region, are often effective in accomplishing the desired result. If all these means fail, the catheter must be used as the last resort. During the entire lying-in the bladder should be emptied every six hours.

Evacuation of the Bowels. – There should be an evacuation of the bowels in from twenty-four to thirty-six hours after the labor. For this purpose a seidlitz powder may be given, or the liquid citrate of magnesia. If this does not suffice, an enema of warm water, to which a little soap or two teaspoonfuls of glycerin have been added, may be given. Two pints of water should be prepared; the patient will retain as much as she comfortably can, and as long as she can. The bowels should be opened daily after the first day.

After-pains are caused by the same physiologic process that causes labor pains— namely, by the contractions of the uterus. After the first confinement the after-pains are, as a rule, not severe; attention to the regular emptying of the bladder and bowels also lessens the severity of the after-pains; these pains seldom last after the second day.

The Lochia. – The discharges of the mother continue for about two weeks, and are called lochia. For the first twenty-four hours they are pure blood; the second and the third day they are of the character of bloody water; from the fourth to the sixth day they have a, greenish-yellow color, and from the tenth to the twelfth day they become pure white. Soiled napkins and dressings should never be allowed to remain in the patient's room.

Duration of the Lying-in. – This lasts for six weeks. During this time the organs of generation are returning to their normal size and condition. In order that the woman may be in the best condition possible at the end of this time, it is essential that for the first two weeks she should remain in bed; and so long as there is any blood in the discharge the woman should not be allowed to sit up. The first sitting up should be in bed, the patient being supported by a bed-rest. During the second two weeks the patient may be allowed to divide her time between the bed and the couch; in the latter part of this time she may be allowed to go around her room a very little; and for two weeks more she should remain on the same floor. The first sitting up should not last more than half an hour. Getting up and going around too soon after the confinement, "being too smart," is one of the most prolific sources of falling of the womb, and all manner of uterine trouble, by which the general health of the woman is greatly impaired.

Lactation.— If it is at all possible, every mother should nurse her own child; in the interests of both the mother and the child. So far as the mother is concerned, the process of lactation is beneficial because it hastens the return of the uterus to its normal size. Wet-nurses are known tyrants, and if the quality of the milk has anything to do with the disposition of the child, as is believed to be the case, the idea is distasteful of having a woman who belongs to the lower classes provide nourishment for your child; and artificial feeding is one unmitigated trouble.

A deficiency of the quantity or the quality of the mother's milk can generally be remedied by the diet and attention to the health of the mother; if the deficiency in quantity persists, the mother's milk can be supplemented by artificial feeding.

There may exist certain conditions of the mother in which nursing her own infant would be inadvisable or even impossible. Syphilis contracted late in the pregnancy, and tuberculosis, are contraindications, owing to the danger of the mother infecting the child. Inversion of the nipples, their excoriation, or persistent sensitiveness may make it impossible. In marked general debility of the mother from any cause whatever, it would be injurious to the mother and the child.

After the mother and the new-born infant have had some hours of rest and sleep, it is advisable to apply the child to the breast, to receive by this first effort the small quantity of milk which is an especial provision to act as a natural purge and to start the bowels of the child into a healthy activity; this also excites the milk glands to secretion. The mother's milk in full supply may be expected in from forty to sixty hours after delivery.

Nursing. — When the mother's nipples are of the normal size and well formed, the healthy infant instinctively suckles at once when placed at the breast, but sometimes it has to be taught; by squeezing out a few drops of milk to wet the nipple, the child will usually take hold, or a little sugar and water may be put on the nipple; a little patience and tact are all that is necessary to insure success. But the infant must be taught to nurse at once before the breasts become engorged with milk.

Under ordinary circumstances the child is to be kept at the breast for one year. But if within this time the menstrual period should recur and be profuse, or should the woman again become pregnant, the quality of the milk becomes poor, and necessitates the immediate weaning of the child; the character of the milk is also altered, and even its secretion may be checked. Nervous agitation may so alter the quality of the milk as to make it poisonous. A fretful temper, fits of anger, grief, and sudden terror not only lessen the quantity of the milk, but render it thin and unhealthful, inducing disturbances of the child's bowels, diarrhea, and so forth.

Position of the Mother When Nursing. — When in bed in the recumbent position, the mother should lie on that side from which the infant is going to nurse; when up, the mother should sit erect.

Care of the Nipples. — Immediately after each nursing the nipples should be washed off in a saturated solution of boric acid in cold water, and dried with a soft cloth. If they are disposed to crack, anoint them with cocoa-butter immediately after each cleansing. If the skin of the nipple is very sensitive, a nipple-shield should be used for the first few days; or should the nipple become sore at any time, the shield can be resorted to. The nipple-shield must fit tightly; the best ones are made of glass with a rubber tip. In the intervals of nursing the nipple-shield should be kept in cold water after it has been thoroughly cleansed by being brushed on both sides.

The breasts are sometimes distended from an over-secretion of milk; this is relieved by saline cathartics, by abstinence from liquids, and by the use of a compression breast bandage. This is made of a straight piece of muslin, with a shallow notch cut in one edge for the neck, and, a deep one for each arm; the bandage is closely applied over the breasts, and the ends pinned in front; it is also pinned over the shoulders.

In debilitated women the supply of milk may be insufficient; the most reliable evidence of this is the fact that the infant ceases to gain in weight.

CHAPTER XIII.

THE NEW-BORN INFANT.

The Infant's Toilet; the Crib; Feeding of Infants; Artificial Feeding; the Wet-nurse; Characteristics of Healthy Infants; the Stools; Constipation; Urination; Dentition.

> "O thou child of many prayers,
> Life hath quicksands; life hath snares."
>
> — LONGFELLOW.

The Infant's Toilet. — So soon as the mother has been made comfortable, the toilet of the infant is attended to. This should be made near the register or stove; and the lap of the nurse should be covered with a small flannel blanket. The baby's body will be found to be covered over with a white, greasy, somewhat cheesy substance; some sort of grease is needed for its removal; rendered lard, sweet oil, and lanolin are the best; vaselin is less effective. All of this cheesy substance must be at once removed; the most difficult parts will be in the folds and creases. The nurse should grease the palms of her hands, then take the head of the child between them, and thoroughly grease it; particular attention must be given to the ears; then come the neck, shoulders, arms, chest and back, groins, external genital organs, and lower extremities. After the child has been thoroughly gone over, the grease should be rubbed off with a soft towel.

A rectal injection of one tablespoonful of warm water is given at once to unload the bowels of the meconium; this generally acts before the baby's toilet is completed. The meconium is the first discharge from the infant's bowels after birth, and that which had collected in the intestines during the pregnancy.

The Baby's Bath. — The baby's bath-tub is filled about one-third full of water at a temperature of 100° F., tested by the thermometer. The baby is then gradually immersed in the water, with the exception of the head; this is supported on the left wrist of the nurse, which passes under the infant's neck, while her hand grasps the left shoulder; with the right hand the nurse quickly rubs over the child's head and body; the entire bath should not occupy over five minutes. The infant is then lifted out into the lap of the nurse, on which is spread a soft, warm towel, with which it is carefully dried. One of the important points in giving the infant its bath is to be sure that the groins, arm-pits, and genitals are thoroughly well dried; otherwise excoriation at these parts is sure to occur.

After this a daily tub-bath is given in the same way; soap is rarely needed; when it is, castile soap should be used; its constant use is not necessary and would only irritate the skin. These daily baths strengthen the nervous system and prevent coughs and colds. The bath should be given during the morning, one hour after feeding, and should not last more than five minutes. The mother herself, just as soon as she is able to go around, should superintend the bath; in this way she is assured that if properly given, and will also recognize any incipient affection of the child. These daily baths should be continued till the child is four years old. Powder is not essential; but if it is desired, a plain talcum powder may be used.

The Dressing of the Cord. — After the bath the ligature which was tied around the cord at the birth of the child will be found slightly loosened; this should first be made tight, and then the cord, doubled back on itself, should be tied by the ends of the same ligature. A square of soft sterilized linen or gauze is slit up to its center; the cord is allowed to pass through this slit, which looks toward the child's right; the stump of cord is laid on the left and the ends of gauze are folded over this; the whole is kept in place by the abdominal bandage. As there is some exudation from the cord, it is necessary to change these dressings twice a day; as this exudation is of a somewhat gluey nature, it will be found that the dressings stick to the cord. In removing the gauze great care must be used not to make any traction on the cord; when the infant is placed in the bath, the water loosens the dressing and it falls off in the water; at other times it must be removed with the greatest care. There should never be any odor about the cord; it usually drops off about the fifth day.

The process of ulceration by which the cord falls off leaves an open surface on the child's body which offers an avenue for septic infection. Great care must therefore be taken that the nurse's hands or anything which comes in contact with this surface should be perfectly clean. The dressings used must be thoroughly antiseptic.

Care should be used not to fasten the abdominal bandage too tightly; the bath is given on an empty stomach, and allowance should be made for this; the binder should be loose enough to allow two or three fingers to easily slip under it.

The Meconium. – The First discharge that comes from the bowels is of a dark, greenish color, and should come away during the first twenty-four hours; if it does not, the baby may suffer a good deal of pain, and an enema of warm water must be given. As this substance is very difficult to be washed out of napkins, the first ones used should be old and afterward be burned.

Cleansing. – Every time the napkin needs to be changed, even if it is only wet, the baby should be washed with warm water. A napkin should never be used twice without washing; it chafes the child, and it is an unsafe as well as a filthy practice; the napkin must always be removed as soon as it is wet.

The Infant's Toilet. – After the application of the binder and napkin, comes the undervest; the fingers of the nurse are passed up through the sleeve to seize the infant's hand and pull it through; as soon as it gets a little older the child will grasp a finger laid in its palm, which greatly facilitates this part of the toilet. The stockings are next put on and pinned with safety-pins to the napkin; then comes the petticoat, the band of which is also loosely fastened with safety-pins, and with the slip the toilet is complete. All the clothing should be changed night and morning.

The eyes and mouth should be washed out with separate pieces of gauze or old linen. For the mouth, a small piece of cloth wet in warm water is wrapped around the little finger of the right hand, going into the left angle of the baby's mouth and coming out at the right, going between the gums and cheeks as well as over the tongue. This procedure should be gone through with every time preceding and following the nursing, and in this way the milk is prevented from souring in the mouth, and the digestion is kept in good condition. A sore mouth in a baby indicates carelessness on the part of the nurse.

A soft hair-brush may be used, but the scalp is too tender to permit the use of a comb.

After the toilet has been completed, the baby is laid in its crib, on the right side of the body, and warmly covered. The weaker the baby, the more attention must be paid to the external warmth. It may be necessary to place a warm-water bottle in the crib, but this must never touch the infant.

The Crib. – The infant must have its own crib, without rockers, and it must on no account be put to sleep in the same bed with its mother. In its early life it should never be taken out of its crib except to be fed, to have its clothing changed, or to be bathed. There should be no holding on the lap, no dangling, no carrying or fussing over the new-born infant; and the more the baby is let alone, the better and healthier it will be. If baby cries, look at once to see if it needs a fresh napkin; if not, if any pins are sticking into it, if the clothing is possibly too tight; if none of these things are wrong, give it a sup of water and turn it over on the other side. The baby often becomes restless by sleeping for several hours in the same position. But on no account take the infant up out of its crib simply because it cries.

Cheerfulness and good nature on the part of the infant are dependent on its general good health. A healthy infant should not have colic, but if such is the case, there is a peculiar look of distress on the face, which indicates that the child is in pain; what is needed is warmth or medication according to the severity of the case, but never floor walking. Begin the latter procedure, and you may hope to keep it up for several years.

Ventilation. – The air is sometimes vitiated for children's uses in various ways; their nervous susceptibilities are greater than those of older people. A very little odor of tobacco may cause nausea and discomfort to an infant in arms. The atmosphere of the room should be sweet and pure and unscented. All scents and perfumes affect the nervous system, and by constant excitation do it damage. A bouquet of flowers renders the air of a closed room too heavy.

Feeding of Infants. – During the day the infant should be put to the breast once every two hours, and once every three hours during the night. This interval of time between the feeding is necessary in order that there may be sufficient time given for digestion to take place. Regurgitation of milk soon after feeding is a sign that the stomach has been overfilled. As the infant usually falls asleep after nursing, it is necessary to waken it up at the time for the next nursing, as good digestion depends upon regularity of feeding.

For the first nursing the infant may be put to the breast in from two to six hours after the labor if the mother is sufficiently rested; from ten to twenty minutes is long enough for each nursing. Before each nursing the nipples should be carefully washed off with a solution of boric acid. The first secretion of the breasts is laxative; that is, it acts on the bowels, and makes is unnecessary to give the infant anything to take for this purpose. The breasts should be used alternately in feeding the infant, as this allows a longer time for the accumulation of the milk. For the first few days the infant needs very little food, and the mother's milk is generally sufficient.

The infant should be given a teaspoonful of cool water to drink two or three times a day, as the milk does not quench the thirst. The water should be sterilized by boiling, and be kept in an air-tight flask.

At the end of the third month the intervals of nursing for the daytime should be three hours, and the last nursing at night should be at eleven o'clock, and the first nursing in the morning at five o'clock; thus allowing the mother an interval of six hours of unbroken sleep.

The best evidence of the proper nutrition of the child is a progressive gain in weight. The child should be weighed every week. A loss of a few ounces usually takes place during the first few days after birth, so that the child does well if at the end of the first week it weighs as much as it did at birth. After the first week the weekly gain should not fall below five ounces.

The Wet-nurse. – When the mother for any reason whatever is not able to nurse her child, the best substitute is a wet-nurse. Before she is employed the wet-nurse should always be carefully examined by a physician to insure her freedom from disease. The best age is between twenty and thirty years, and the age of the child of the nurse should be at least within a month of that of the child to be nursed. The best sign of the good health of the nurse and of the condition of her milk is furnished by the health of her own child. The breasts should be well formed and the nipple of good shape. It is well, if possible, to get a woman who has borne several children, as she will understand the care of the child better. No woman who is not perfectly healthy is fit to be a wet-nurse; and even after she has been engaged her health and her habits must be watched over.

Artificial Feeding. — The first requisite in artificial feeding is that the milk shall be made to correspond as nearly as possible to that of the mother. For this purpose the following formula, prepared by Rotch, of modified cow's milk is considered the best:

Milk	2 ounces
Cream	3 ounces
Water	10 drams
Milk-sugar	6 3/4 drams
Lime-water	1 ounce

To make one pint of the mixture for use in the twenty-four hours, take the milk and cream as soon as it comes in the morning, and mix as above directed.

No less important than the correct proportions of the ingredients, is freedom from disease germs and bacteria of putrefaction. Complete sterilization is possible by prolonged boiling; but experience has proved that under prolonged exposure to a temperature near the boiling-point certain changes take place in the albuminoids of the milk which greatly impair its digestibility. Full sterilization of milk for infant feeding has therefore practically been abandoned. It has been found that milk heated to 167° F. for twenty minutes, and promptly chilled by placing on ice, remains practically sterile for twenty-four hours, and it is spared the injurious changes which take place at a higher temperature. This process is known as Pasteurization. The Arnold steam sterilizer affords a convenient method of sterilizing; if used with the cover removed, the steam chamber being open, the temperature of the steam chamber does not exceed 170° F.

It is claimed that in the Arnold steam sterilizer, with the use of a suitable gas stove, the water begins to boil at the end of two minutes after the gas is lighted. A four-ounce bottle of milk at an initial temperature of 70° F. in the open steam chamber attains a temperature of 170° in just one hour. An exposure of about one hour and twenty minutes in the steam chamber is therefore necessary for the Pasteurization.

The rules for sterilizing are as follows:

First, clean the bottles thoroughly; then place them in cold water, which is allowed to come to boil and boiled for ten minutes.

Second, fill each with the milk you wish to use; put in the rubber cork without the glass plug; this leaves a small opening in the rubber cork; set the bottle in the basket, then in the boiler.

Third, set in the refrigerator until needed for use.

Fourth, when wanted for use, place a bottle of the milk so prepared in the tin mug which accompanies the sterilizer; fill the mug with hot water to the height of the milk in the bottle, heat the milk to the temperature of 99° F., remove the rubber cork and put on the nipple, when it is ready for use.

Fifth, cleanse the bottle immediately after using; throw away any milk that has not been used.

Sixth, if the steaming process is preferred, place the basket without the bottles in the boiler, fill the water up to, but not above, the bottom of the basket, place the bottles in the basket, and proceed as before.

It is important that the milk should be sterilized or Pasteurized as soon as it is served in the morning. Each bottle must be thoroughly washed as soon as it is emptied. Milk sterilized in this way will keep for days without spoiling, as it is hermetically sealed and all the unhealthy germs have been removed.

The most exact method for the artificial feeding of infants, and that which most nearly approaches the mother's milk, is that used by the "Walker-Gordon Laboratory," branches of which are to be found in many of the large cities.

Not only is the greatest care taken that the milk used shall be pure and sterilized ready for use, but these laboratories are equipped by special machinery which separates the important elements of the milk — namely, the fat, the milk-sugar, and the proteids. So that the physician can modify the proportions of these various ingredients of the milk to meet the necessity of the age and requirements of the infant.

When the milk contains too little sugar, the infant does not gain as rapidly in weight as it would otherwise do. Too much sugar in the milk is indicated by colic, thin, green, or acid stools, or eructations of gas from the stomach.

An excess of fat in the milk is indicated by vomiting; too little fat causes constipation with dry hard stools. Proteids in excess are a prolific cause of colic and also of diarrhea.

Prescription blanks are furnished the physician, who fills out the percentages of fat, milk-sugar, proteids, and alkalinity, to suit the age, weight, and general condition of the child. He orders also the amount to be given at each feeding, and the number of feedings to be given in the twenty-four hours. Each bottle contains just the amount to be given at one feeding. All that the mother needs to do is to place the bottle in a receptacle containing warm water, until the milk has attained a temperature of 99° F., remove the cotton stopper, and put on the nipple, when it is ready for use.

The Nursing Bottle. — This should be of clear glass, with a rounded bottom, and of such a shape as is easy to clean; so that no particles will cling around a corner which cannot be reached. The graduated bottle is the most convenient, as it enables the quantities of each of the materials used in the preparation of the feeding to be mixed in the bottle, doing away with the trouble of measuring before putting into the bottle.

Rubber Nipples. — Two nipples should be kept for alternate use, and no nipple should be used longer than two weeks. A soft rubber of conical shape is best, with an opening at the top which is not too large, so that the milk will not flow through, as it is desirable that the child should obtain the milk by suction. So soon as the feeding is over, the nipple should be removed from the bottle, and brushed on both sides with a stiff brush. It should then be put in cold water, where it is kept until it is again wanted.

The baby should be fed slowly, from ten to twenty minutes being taken for each feeding. Sucking from an empty bottle or with a nipple in the mouth should never be permitted, as in this way the baby draws air into its stomach, which will result in colic. Each flask should contain only enough for one feeding.

In lieu of the regular sterilizing apparatus, milk may be similarly prepared by placing the milk in an ordinary glass fruit-jar with a screw lid. This is placed in a colander over a pot of boiling water; the milk should be allowed to boil in the open jar for two minutes; the jar-lid is then screwed on, and it should steam for twenty minutes longer.

The capacity of the infant stomach at birth is about one ounce, which is the average quantity of food that should be taken at one meal. The average rate of increase in the amount of food is one and a half drams a week for the first six months; subsequently somewhat less. The intervals of feeding should be two hours at birth, and increased to three hours at the end of the third month. The food should be given at a temperature of 99° F. and fed directly from the sterilizing bottle.

Fresh Air.— In warm weather the baby is taken out-of-doors in from three to four weeks after birth; in cold weather not before two to three months. In the latter case it is prepared for the change by being first dressed as for the street, with wrap and cap; the windows of the room are then opened, and the infant is carried about here. In the winter months when the baby is first taken out, it is better to carry it in the arms, as it will be kept warmer in this way, and if it does become chilled it will be more quickly noticed.

Characteristics of the Healthy Infant.— The average weight of an infant at birth is about seven pounds, and its length is about twenty inches; the extremes are four pounds or a little less up to eleven pounds. The head and trunk of the child are developed out of proportion to the limbs.

The skin of the new-born infant varies from pinkish to red; about the fourth day the color becomes somewhat yellowish; this tinge should disappear about the end of the second week, and at the same time the skin begins to peel off. This process lasts about two weeks longer, when the baby's skin takes on its normal color.

The shape of the head varies greatly, much being due to the amount of pressure during labor; but this disappears in a few days. As a rule, the large bones of the head are felt to be separated by membranous ridges called sutures; there is one on the median line on the top of the head, and at either end of the suture is a large open space, called a fontanel. The largest one is at the front of the head, and is called the anterior fontanel; it is about large enough to be covered by the tips of two fingers, and is of a lozenge shape; this opening does not close till the child is about eighteen months old. In a healthy baby this fontanel should be on a level with the bones of the head; a slight pulsation may be noticed in it, due to the pulsations of the vessels of the brain. There is a much smaller three-cornered fontanel at the back of the suture, and one behind either ear; these soon close up with bone.

A new-born baby cannot probably do any more than distinguish light from darkness. Up to the sixth week there is an inability at coordination of the ocular muscles; after this time the eyes begin to move in an orderly manner, and they will follow a bright object moved slowly in front of them. At about the end of the second month rapid movements are perceived, as is evinced by the child's closing its eyes quickly on an object suddenly approaching it. At three months the child begins to recognize colors; the first recognized are yellow, red, pure white, gray, and black. But the faculty of distinguishing between colors is not perfected till the third year. The mother is recognized about the third month. Hearing and a sense of smell develop rapidly after birth; loud noises in its vicinity will cause a child to start during the first day after birth. By the time the child has reached three months of age it shows signs of having a mind of its own, and is capable of exercising thought. It grasps for objects, and indicates its likes and dislikes. At from eight to ten months it can utter several syllables, and at the age of one year should be able to say mama and papa; at two years it should be able to frame short sentences.

Weight of the Baby. — By the end of the sixth month the child's weight should be double what it was at birth; that is, about fourteen pounds; at the end of the twelfth month be three times as much as at birth, or about twenty pounds.

Muscular Action. — Muscular action in the new-born infant is entirely involuntary, there being no voluntary acts until about the end of the third month. Sucking and licking are largely instinctive. The movements of the arms and legs are impulsive acts, and occur during sleep, just as they did in the intra-uterine life. The act of raising the head, which is attempted about the fourth month in healthy children, is volitional, requiring not so much added strength of muscle as power of coordination. As volition develops the power of coordination gradually increases, and the child learns to perform voluntary or purposeful acts. Voluntary grasping is done after the fourth month. As the child learns to balance its head, it attempts to sit up. This act is not successfully accomplished until about the fortieth week; the child sits firmly alone when ten or eleven months old. Before this time it is necessary to support the head and spine of the child with the hand. By the third or fourth month the infant should be able to grasp things. The child begins to creep about the ninth month. The clothing should be so arranged as to allow entire freedom of motion.

It should be able to stand up by a chair by the tenth month, and be able to walk alone at the end of the first year. It is important that parents should know this, since not knowing what a normal baby ought to be able to do, cases of birth palsy, or even an attack of paralysis due to teething, are not infrequently overlooked, not only by the mother, but even by the doctor, who attributes the inability of the child to do what other children can do at this age simply to weakness, which the child will outgrow; and thus the time passes in which the most could be done to cure the child and to prevent the subsequent deformity.

A baby should not be forced to stand or walk; a very stout baby, on account of its weight, will stand up and walk much later than a slight one, the two being equally healthy. Or if a baby has been sick, it will feel no inclination to stand up. Naturally, a child creeps before it walks, and this develops the muscles of the lower limbs, so that they will support the weight of the child in standing. By prematurely forcing a child to stand up and walk, there is danger of causing bow-legs, as the bones of the legs are still weak; the child should be discouraged from standing up too much rather than encouraged to stand up more.

Sleep. – A large proportion of the time of early infancy is spent in sleep; for the first few weeks the infant only wakens up to be fed. During sleep the eyelids should be tightly closed; a partial opening of the lids, showing the whites of the eyes, is an indication of ill health. Up to the age of six, children require twelve hours of sleep at night, besides an hour or more in the middle of the day; the child should be permitted to sleep as long in the morning as it will.

Respiration. – The healthy infant breathes on an average forty-four times a minute; the only time the respirations can be satisfactorily counted is during sleep. When the child is awake, the respirations are hurried by slight movements of the body, crying, and so forth. The average pulse of a newborn baby is one hundred and forty; this is hurried by the same causes that hastens respirations; the pulse is most easily counted at the anterior fontanel. The average temperature of the infant is 99° F. When the tip of the nose and the extremities are cold, it indicates a lowered vitality.

The nature of the child's cry indicates, variously, hunger, temper, or pain; the mother will soon learn to distinguish these varieties. If the child cries because it is hungry, the cry ceases so soon as it is fed. But a child is never to be fed simply because it cries; it must be fed on the hour by the clock. If this rule is not strictly adhered to, it will suffer all the forms of indigestion and colic that babies are heir to. If it cries because of colic, there is a drawn look on the face, and at the same time the legs are sharply flexed on the thighs and the thighs on the abdomen. If the cries are due to earache, the head will be rolled about from one side to the other. In either case nothing will stop the cries until the pain is relieved. A baby does not shed tears until the third month.

The Stools. – The stools of a very young baby fed on breast-milk should be of a yellow or orange color. There should be three or four evacuations daily; they should contain no curds. Stools of bottle-fed babies are lighter in color and more offensive.

Constipation. — Constipation is not uncommon in infancy; it may be overcome by the use of a soap suppository, or by an injection of warm soap-suds into the bowel, or by an injection of oil and water, or by gentle friction over the bowel, following the course of the large intestine.

To make the soap suppository, take a piece of castile soap about an inch long, give it the shape of a cone not any larger than the end of the little finger, and make it perfectly smooth. This is inserted to about half of its length into the rectum and held there until it causes the bowels to move.

The bowel injection is best given by means of the single-bulb syringe, known as the eye and ear syringe; the bulb holds about two tablespoonfuls of liquid. This may be warm cotton-seed oil, sweet oil, or glycerin one teaspoonful to warm water two tablespoonfuls. The nozle should be small, smooth, and well oiled. It should be very carefully introduced into the bowel, being directed a little to the left side, and the bulb gently squeezed to force the contents into the bowel. The injection is more effective if it is retained for a little while; this is accomplished by making slight pressure on the anus with a towel.

Rubbing the abdomen for about ten minutes in the direction of the large bowel is sometimes very effective in overcoming constipation; begin in the right groin and rub up as far as the border of the ribs, then across to the left, then down on the left side.

Vomiting. — Vomiting means often only that the stomach has been overfilled, and may be relieved by withholding all food for a few hours.

Urination. — The frequency of urination in a newborn baby will vary greatly with the weather and other conditions; in cool weather it is not unusual for the napkin to need changing almost every hour. Healthy urine should not stain the napkin. The new-born infant secretes very little urine until it begins to take nourishment freely. The bladder is usually emptied during birth, and very often the bowels also, so that if the child seems well and there is no malformation of the parts, the family may be assured that the apparent retention of urine is only temporary.

The use of hot fomentations over the kidneys and bladder will often hasten the evacuation of urine if it has been unduly delayed. If the secretion seems highly concentrated, a drop of sweet spirits of niter in a teaspoonful of water may be given every two hours.

Teething. — The first tooth generally appears about the end of the fourth month; in delicate children they come later. As a rule, the lower front teeth come first, coming in pairs, one tooth coming on each side of the mouth; followed in about a month by the corresponding teeth in the upper jaw. Preceding their appearance the gums become swollen, hot, and painful, and the saliva forms in excess and runs from the mouth. The child is irritable, flushed and restless; and there usually occurs some disturbance of the bowels, commonly diarrhea. This all indicates a nervous derangement, and calls for a judicious diet and general careful oversight. The symptoms subside when the teeth are through. During teething the child manifests a desire to bite on something, and a soft rubber ring will give it great comfort.

The first set of teeth are twenty in number, and are usually cut in groups, starting about the fourth month and continuing until between the twentieth and thirtieth month, when the first dentition should be complete. As a rule there is an interval of rest between the eruption of the various groups. During dentition children are generally more peevish and fretful than usual, but there should be no general constitutional disturbance. During dentition it is of especial importance to keep the bowels well opened; it is better to have them too loose than costive; constipation at this time greatly increases the tendency to convulsions.

Bottle-fed babies are apt to cut their teeth later than those nursed at the breast. The lack of appearance of any teeth before the end of the first year indicates that the nutrition of the child is below par, or, in other words, that the child has rickets. The permanent teeth begin to appear about the sixth or seventh year.

PART IV.— THE MENOPAUSE.

CHAPTER XIV.

THE MENOPAUSE.

Average Duration of the Menstrual Function; Duration of Menopause; the Menopause; General Phenomena of the Menopause; Prominent Symptoms of Menopause; Pathologic Conditions of the Menopause; Hemorrhage at the Menopause a Significant Symptom of Cancer; Causes of Suffering at Menopause.

> "Yet I doubt not through the ages one increasing purpose runs,
> And the thoughts of men are widened with the process of the suns.
> Knowledge comes, but wisdom lingers, and I linger on the shore,
> And the individual withers, and the world is more and more.
> Knowledge comes, but wisdom lingers, and he bears a laden breast,
> Full of sad experience, moving toward the stillness of his rest."
>
> — *"Locksley Hall."*

Average Duration of Menstrual Function.— The average duration of the menstrual function is from thirty to thirty-two years. Raciborski estimated the duration of menstrual life at about thirty-one years and nine months. According to him, the mean age of puberty at Paris was fourteen years and seven months; therefore, the average age of the menopause was forty-six and one-half years. Tilt gives the average age of the cessation of menstruation in 1082 cases as forty-five years and nine months. The average age is between forty-five and fifty years. It has been shown by Krieger, Kisch, and others, that the earlier the menses appear, the later they cease, and vice versa. However, when the first period is unusually early or late, the menopause comes very early. Also that the sexual function is usually abolished earlier in the laboring classes, who are compelled to work hard and who have many cares, than in the well-to-do and rich.

Race does unquestionably influence the duration, but given a sound healthy race, which is not too much enervated with civilization, and the menstrual process will, equally with the total physical vigor and the vitality, be increased. At the present day there is an increased sexual vitality, which shows itself in the fact that the duration of menstrual life has been increased three to four years during the past generation. The inference can be fairly deduced that vigorous vitality causes prolongation of the menstrual process and the actual age.

Duration of Menopause.— By the menopause or climacteric is understood the whole period from the beginning irregularities in the time of appearance of the menstrual flow until its actual cessation. The average duration of the menopause is from two and a half to three years.

The Menopause.— The menopause is a physiologic and conservative process. It occurs at a time of life when all the tissues are most stable and the nutrition of the body is at its best. Other physiologic changes which occur at the same time are decrease in the size of the spleen and lymphatic glands, the muscular coats of the intestine atrophy, and lessened peristalsis ensues; hence the increased tendency to constipation. These are not the degenerations of age, but the blood-supplying, blood-making, and blood-elaborating organs of the body have completed the growth of the organism, done their work, and are striking a balance with the needs of the economy.

The object of each metamorphic or developmental epoch is a critical readjustment of the organism, in order to insure the greatest possible amount of health for each subsequent period of life. In the vast majority of cases this object is quietly effected, but sometimes the constitution only rallies after having been severely shaken for a varying period.

General Phenomena of the Menopause.— Borner states that while many women pass this period without noting any change in their former condition, and are conscious of the occurrence of the change of life only by reason of the absence of the menstrual flow, others suffer for years with a host of troubles.

One of the most essential changes is that of the woman s psychic condition— from slight vagaries, loss of interest in the daily affairs of life, to melancholia and insanity.

"Two factors are generally taken into account: first, the sudden cessation of the menses; second, the reflections of the patient caused by her condition, meditations on the loss of youth and sexual power, and anxiety in view of the dangers of the climacteric. It cannot be denied that there is some truth in the supposed sad thoughts about the beginning of old age, and the depression caused by them can scarcely be considered abnormal" (Borner).

Napier believes that it is extremely rare for the cessation to occur without some physical discomfort or some disturbance of the nervous system, but adds that: "Some women, however, cease menstruating with very slight inconvenience." As a rule, the woman misses one, two, or more periods, then a menstruation of almost normal quantity and duration; and this is again repeated at gradually longer intervals, and with a diminished flow, until actual cessation occurs.

The periods cease owing to the degeneration and disappearance of the glandular tissues of the uterus, and secondarily to similar changes in the ovaries and other glands. This is followed by an atrophy of all the structures of the genitalia.

An increase in the size of the uterus, from increase in the amount of blood, is frequently noticed at the beginning of the menopause; later it becomes smaller in all its dimensions. The wall becomes thinner; the cervix becomes shorter and thinner, sometimes hard, sometimes flabby as a membrane. But the distinguishing feature of the menopastic uterus is atrophy of its lining membrane.

The changes in the uterus and Fallopian tubes are earlier than those in the ovaries, so that ovulation, though lessened in activity, may persist for a considerable time after menstruation has ceased. Ovarian atrophy has been referred to senile rather than menopastic changes.

Atrophy of the ovaries occurs very gradually. Peuch found that in one case the ovaries were of normal size three years after the establishment of the menopause. Kiwisch describes the structural change in this gland as consisting, on the one hand, of an increase of the connective-tissue stroma; and, on the other hand, the Graafian vesicles themselves undergo retrograde change. In consequence of these microscopic changes, which take place very slowly, the entire organ becomes harder and smaller.

Napier believes that the ovaries secrete specialized substances which aid in determining menstruation; and that in a less degree the utricular glands and the glands of the Fallopian tubes share in this action. He considers that this is probably secondary to the chain of peripheral irritation from the uterine glands, but that this secretion is none the less an essential feature of the menstrual process.

In support of this view he calls attention to the pigmentation of the skin which occurs during pregnancy and chlorosis, showing that the absence of the catamenia results in the retention in the blood of some substance which would normally be excreted at this time.

Other atrophic changes in the genitalia are shriveling of the vulva, with prolapse of the vagina or uterus from relaxation of the ligaments and loss of the natural support afforded by the changed perineal body.

Uterine catarrh occurs almost invariably, and only ceases in advanced years. Displacements of all kinds are frequent, but on account of the now greatly diminished weight of the uterus, these are insignificant.

The vagina is at first almost always hyperemic, but this disappears as the vessels successively atrophy. The vagina gradually becomes narrower and shorter. The mucous membrane loses its rugae and presents a pale, grayish, blanched hue.

The researches of Byron Robinson, made by the dissection of a number of old women, show that after the menopause not only is there an atrophy of the genital organs, but that the hypogastric plexus of the great sympathetic nervous system also shrinks away. "It becomes smaller and firmer, and no doubt some strands disappear. On this fact must he based the pathologic symptoms accompanying the cessation of the menstrual function."

The importance of the genital organs is shown by the vast nerve-supply sent to them. When this great nerve-tract becomes atrophic, so that it can no longer transmit the higher physiologic orders, all parts of the sympathetic system must be unbalanced, until a new line, the next line of least resistance is established. And Robinson believes that this is the explanation of the many pathologic manifestations of every viscus at the menopause; that is, "the irritation which arises by trying to pass more nervous impulses over plexuses than normal gives origin to what is unfortunately known as functional disease. It is just as organic as any disease, only we are unable to detect it."

Chemical changes in the blood and tissues are constant vital phenomena; increased oxidation causes increased activity of the circulation, increase of temperature, increase of urea and carbonic acid in the economy from retrograde changes, and, finally, during menstrual life the flow of blood from the uterus carried off the effete materials from the highly charged system.

The elimination of albuminoids, as shown by the altered condition of the blood after menstruation, is greater than can be accounted for by the blood discharged. When the menopause is attained suddenly, the retention of such albuminoid substances must act toxically. Hence the resulting clinical fact that sudden cessation of the menses is, in the majority of cases, attended with pronounced symptoms of discomfort, and it is in these cases that untoward results are most likely.

James Oliver believes that the catamenial flow eliminates from the body substances whose presence in the blood would exert a deleterious influence on the animal economy.

The Prominent Symptoms of the Menopause.— Christopher Martin holds that the symptoms of the change of life are produced largely by a condition of instability and increased excitability of certain other cerebrospinal centers directly brought about by failure of the menstrual center, and adds: "It is probable that the ovaries, like the liver and thyroid gland, modify the blood circulating through them, and add to the blood some peculiar product of their metabolism. It may be that some of the climacteric symptoms are due to the loss of this substance from the system."

Arthur Johnstone's theory of the symptoms of the menopause is that the lining membrane of the uterus atrophies and becomes old cicatricial tissue, and sinks into quiet decay. The nervous system begins to readjust itself; but no longer having free outlet through the soft, lymphoid tissues of the uterus, the wave pressure meets with resistance and a choppy sea results. Vertigos, bilious attacks, and so forth are nothing more than reflex waves. The weakest organ of the individual is the one that generally suffers. And that the kidneys, which all along have borne the brunt of life, should now show positive signs of disease is natural.

The etiology and pathology of the menopause lie in the sympathetic nervous system. And it is by the breaking up of the harmony of previous processes that nervous disturbances are produced.

After the cessation of the flow, over 8% of women suffer from "flashes"; this symptom is caused by irritation of the heart and vasomotor centers. The blood-vessels of the head and neck seem to be most affected, yet the skin of the whole body shares in the disturbance. Besides the vasomotor and heat center being disturbed, the sweat center is irritated. The flushes and flashes are followed by various degrees of sweating, which varies from a slight moisture to great drops.

Nervous irritability is a prominent symptom in 8% of women at the time of the menopause. Most of the pain arises around the stomach; that is, the solar plexus. Digestive disturbances are very common at this time; they may be in the shape of fermentation, diarrhea, or constipation, accompanied by congestion of the liver.

Tilt holds the very plausible view that the too strong reaction of the sexual organs on the central ganglia of the sympathetic nervous system is their principal cause of disease. Puberty, menstruation, pregnancy, lactation, or the menopause almost always entail some derangement of this system which is sometimes sufficiently severe to lead to insanity and suicide. Debility underlies all affections of the sympathetic nervous system, in the same way as nervous irritability underlies all cerebral diseases. Sometimes there is an overpowering sense of exhaustion pervading the whole system.

Forms of climacteric insanity are delirium, mania, hypochondriasis, melancholia, irresponsible impulses, and the perversion of moral instincts.

"If the reproductive apparatus does not act on the brain by the instrumentality of the circulating organs of the blood, it must do so by means of the nerves. The genital apparatus is richly endowed with nerves from the sympathetic system, and I have shown how frequently evident signs of disturbance in these centers coincided or alternated with headaches, nervousness, hysteria, and epilepsy. What wonder, then, if the same powerful influence of the sexual organs, through the instrumentality of the sympathetic system, should at times produce a permanent derangement of the mental and moral faculties. I am thus led to look on the sympathetic nervous center as a source of vital power producing reflex morbid phenomena, in accordance with variable cerebral predisposition" (Tilt).

Another very frequent symptom of the menopause is distress in the region of the heart, with palpitation and shortness of breath. It may be caused by the condition of the blood, whether it be impoverished — anemia — or too rich in red globules; by reflex irritation of the pneumogastric or sympathetic nerves; by overexertion; or by alcoholism. It may also be due to general debility; the woman resists fatigue less easily, and she experiences a general malaise. To the palpitations are rapidly added faintness and shortness of breath. The sleep is troubled with distress in the region of the heart. It is said that women in whom the menopause occurs early are more liable to tachycardia than those who menstruate later in life; and that it occurs with especial frequency when the menopause has been prematurely induced by surgical operation or by disease. It is believed that this functional heart trouble is caused by the increased connective-tissue fibers of the sexual organs acting in some unknown way on the terminal fibers of the sympathetic; and it is not infrequently due to the formation of scar tissue at the seat of a cervical laceration, and has often been promptly and permanently relieved by removing the cicatricial tissue and suturing the wound. The cause acts by producing a transitory paralysis of the inhibitory fibers of the pneumogastric nerve.

Pathologic Conditions of the Menopause.— Perhaps the most alarming symptom of the menopause is *hemorrhage*. It may be due to general or local causes. Among the general causes are diseases of the heart, lungs, spleen, and kidneys. Local causes of hemorrhage are: inflammation of the lining membrane of the uterus, chronic pelvic inflammations, faulty uterine positions, erosions and ulcerations of the mouth of the uterus, fibroid tumors, and cancer. All competent observers agree that cancer in women is much commoner from forty to fifty years than at any other age.

Hemorrhages occupy the foremost place among the pathologic phenomena of the genital tract during the menopause. Hemorrhage has been attributed in many instances to the senile rigidity and friability of the uterine vessels, which are not in a condition to offer sufficient resistance to the blood-pressure which is brought to bear on their walls; there is also softening and relaxation of the uterine tissue. Additional causes are found in the circulatory disturbances in the pelvic organs, whereby the outflow of blood from the pelvic vessels is hindered a chronic congestion in the uterine vessels is produced. It has also been attributed to early and profuse menstruation, frequent and difficult labors, frequent abortions, and excess in drinking.

The third and last variety includes those cases which may be referred to some disease of the pelvic organs themselves. Anatomic changes may lead up to pathologic conditions. A chief feature characteristic of uterine disease is malnutrition from atrophy— a sudden curtailing of the blood-supply from the degeneration of the genital-nerve apparatus and consequent impaired vitality of tissue from defective nourishment. The anatomic changes in the glands and substance of the uterus also favor the irritation, and the development of new growths, which may be malignant or benign— as cancers, fibroid growths, and so forth.

Hemorrhage at the Menopause a Significant Symptom of Cancer.— Not only should any excessive and prolonged bleeding at the time of the menopause be a source of great anxiety to the woman, but even the irregular appearance of a slight show of blood just sufficient to keep the clothing stained, or a slight bleeding following coition; since all of these are symptoms of very great gravity, and demand an immediate local examination and appropriate treatment.

The widespread belief among the laity that hemorrhage at the time of the menopause is a normal condition, and that if left alone it will stop in the course of a few years, is most erroneous and fatal. On this altar of ignorance thousands of women sacrifice their lives every year. The case-book of any gynecologist will testify to the truth of this statement. The following three cases will serve to illustrate different types of hemorrhage in cancer patients, in no one of which did the patient even suspect that she was suffering from anything more serious than the "vagaries of the menopause."

Case I.— Woman aged seventy years; came on account of incontinence of urine, which had been troublesome for two years. The menopause occurred at fifty. She stated that three or four years previous to her visit, she had had a return of the flow of blood, perhaps twice in the first year, and that during the past year there had been a flow every month— about the same that there used to be. This she took to be a return of the menstrual period. She said, further, that there was a constant bleeding— enough to necessitate the wearing of a napkin— and an occasional severe hemorrhage; that she could not take long walks or drives because of the excessive flow which followed.

The case was one of cancer of the uterus which had spread to all the pelvic viscera; and in addition to this, the patient's general condition was such that any operation was out of the question. Yet the patient had never thought of the possibility of any uterine trouble sufficiently serious to make a local examination necessary. It was only the loss of control over the bladder that drove her to seek a physician's advice.

Case II.— Woman aged fifty-three years came to consult me because of pain, hemorrhage, and loss of weight. There had never been any cessation of the menstrual period. She said that she began to have irregular hemorrhages three years previously, and that they were constantly becoming more frequent and more alarming, and that, in addition to this, there was a constant discharge of blood, which necessitated her wearing a napkin all the time. She also stated that for the preceding six months the pain had been so severe that she had not had one solid night's sleep, and that in that time she had lost forty pounds in weight.

This patient was in the very last stages of cancer of the uterus, and all that could be done for her was to make her comfortable. She had given birth to one child which caused a deep tear of the neck of the womb; and it is probable that this neglected tear was the primary cause of the cancer, which began in the neck of the womb.

Case III. — Woman aged forty-five years; married, but had never had any children. She said that the periods were normal as to duration and amount, but that for the past two years they had two days ahead of time, and that for the past four months she had been having just enough irregular bleeding between the periods to keep her clothing stained.

On examination a diagnosis of cancer of the uterus was made. The pathological examination proved this to be a most malignant type of cancer of the neck of the womb. The entire uterus and appendages were at once removed. And although the patient made an excellent recovery from the operation, she succumbed to the disease one year after the operation was performed.

These cases have been cited at length because they are all typical and because of the variety of symptoms and the great difference of age. Only in one of the cases was there any very severe pain, and it was really the pain, which had become unendurable, which caused the patient to seek relief.

It is the concensus of opinion of the medical profession that cancer of the uterus is one of the common causes of death among women; that the cancer rate of mortality has increased during the last four decades; that it is most common near the time of the menopause; and that there is a direct causal relation between cancer of the neck of the womb and the traumatisms which occur during childbirth.

The symptoms of cancer of the uterus are hemorrhage, a more or less offensive discharge, and pain. The quantity of blood may vary from a slight amount which occasionally stains the clothing to a profuse hemorrhage. In the married, bleeding following coition is always a suggestive symptom. During the menopause any irregular or profuse bleeding should excite suspicion. After the cessation of the menopause any bleeding whatsoever, whether slight or profuse, should always be regarded as a danger signal which demands an immediate and thorough local examination. The same is true of any offensive vaginal discharge. Pain is frequently so late a symptom that to wait for its appearance means that the favorable time to perform an operation has passed by. Emaciation is also a symptom of *advanced* disease.

Cancer is chiefly a disease of the climacteric; when there is a diminished power on the part of the tissues to resist adverse influence. It affects the debilitated and overworked, but it is also found in the well nourished and in the comparatively young.

Cancer always begins as a *local* disease, and when it occurs in the uterus, it is easily accessible and eradicable in its earliest stages; that is, if the disease is discovered in its incipiency, an operation will remove all the diseased tissue. If, on the contrary, the disease is left to nature, the growth spreads out into the surrounding viscera like the roots of a tree in the earth, and the cancer may be literally said to eat into the tissues which it invades. At the same time the germs of the disease begin to be carried all through the body, and the entire constitution is affected.

Prophylaxis, or the Prevention of Cancer. — All pelvic inflammations should be promptly treated, and not allowed to become chronic. Leucorrhea is a symptom of inflammation, the true cause of which can be determined only by local examination. Women who have given birth to children— and this is more especially necessary as they near the age of forty years— should be carefully examined for tears of the neck of the womb. If these tears are extensive they should be repaired, as it is certain that malignant growths frequently do follow local injuries and traumatisms.

Any irregular or profuse bleeding demands an immediate investigation by means of a local examination.

A stormy, irregular, or delayed menopause should excite in the woman a suspicion of some abnormal condition.

The importance of women being carefully watched by gynecologists at this period of their lives cannot be too emphatically stated, for upon the early recognition of cancer depends the only hope of radical cure of the disease. It is estimated that at the present time not less than 95 per cent. of all cases of cancer of the uterus come under the observation of the profession at a stage of the disease when all prospect of permanent relief is out of the question.

It is a deplorable state of affairs that women, not knowing what a normal climacteric is, attribute all hemorrhages, no matter how severe, to the change of life. Therefore, regarding the hemorrhage as a necessary evil, they fail to consult a specialist until the favorable time for eradicating the disease by means of an operation has passed. And whatever knowledge science may bring in the future as to the cure of cancer, at present it is a fact universally agreed upon that early operation, while the cancer is still local, is the only radical cure for the disease.

Pruritus Vulvae. Perhaps one of the most annoying and obstinate symptoms of the menopause is *pruritus vulvae*. This is sometimes caused by sugar in the urine; there is a congestion of the liver which results in sugar being thrown into the system and this is eliminated by the kidneys. It is quite possible that this is due to the altered circulatory conditions of the menopause.

Kidney Disease. — The last pathologic condition which we will mention is *kidney disease.* Le Gendre believes that the menopause exerts a deleterious effect on the kidneys, whether this be a congestion, followed by a diminution in the quantity of urine, or a sort of auto-intoxication due to the retention of a poison in the system that has been prevented from leaving by the ordinary path.

Armstrong says that in almost all cases at the time of the menopause the amount of urine passed is below normal, the specific gravity is increased, and that the urine contains urates and almost always uric acid in excess. Further, that the functions of digestion and assimilation and the various metabolic changes are so largely under the control of the nerve-centers that nothing seems more likely than that so great a disturbance of that system as takes place at the menopause should cause secondary derangements of these most important functions. That being so, the blood becomes loaded with waste products, and the usual symptoms follow — gout and so forth.

It has been a grave question in the mind of the medical profession whether the dangers that certainly do attend the menopause are natural or acquired; that is, could these dangers be averted by any precautions or hygienic measures on the part of women, or are these dangers a necessary accompaniment of this period of life?

Tilt has reached the conclusion that: "The best way to avoid the dangers of this critical time is to meet its approach with a healthy constitution. A marked want of strength prevents the regular succession of the vital phenomena by which all critical periods are carried on. And as the change of life is marked by debility, when this is grafted on constitutional weakness, loss of power will be of long duration. All complaints remain chronic because there is not stamina enough to carry them through their stages."

Causes of Suffering at Menopause.— Dusourd, whose practice lay in an agricultural district in the south of France, as well as Tilt, believes that peasant women suffer little at this time. Their health is generally good when the menopause comes on and they are little liable to nervous disorders. The poor of large towns suffer much at this epoch— the necessity of working hard, the anxieties of poverty and their unhygienic surroundings. But by a fortunate compensation the necessity for working hard prevents or cures the nervous affections which so often assail the rich at this period.

Tilt's cases showed that women who suffered much at the menopause had previously suffered at puberty and at the menstrual periods. And among thirty-nine cases where there was no suffering at the menopause, there was the same immunity from suffering at puberty and at the menstrual epochs.

Tilt's statistics were, or course, taken from English women. In forty-four cases of my own, all women past the menopause, the average age of the first menstruation was fourteen years and four months; and the average age of the actual cessation of the menstrual flow was forty-eight years and five and two-thirds months. Subtracting from this the average age of the first menstruation, we have as the mean age of menstrual life thirty-four years one and two-thirds months; that is, the average duration of the menstrual function was from two to four years longer than that usually given.

A further investigation in order to ascertain any possible relation between the age of marriage and the number of pregnancies and the sufferings of the menopause elicited the following statistics. The average age of marriage was twenty-five years and ten months. Of the four women who were married after thirty-eight years, all were sterile; among the remaining there was an average of slightly above three children each. Forty per cent. of all these cases had one or more miscarriages. Nine had habitually suffered from severe dysmenorrhea, eleven had slight dysmenorrhea, and twenty-two had never felt the slightest inconvenience.

In a list of fifty-two cases, eight were added to the list already given, all of whom had passed the menopause. Five were perfectly healthy and had never suffered the slightest inconvenience. Of these, one was single and only one had one miscarriage. Ten had suffered at the time of the menopause from slight malaise, but not sufficiently to call in a medical attendant. Thirty-seven were more or less seriously ill; thirty of these needed local as well as constitutional treatment, and seven constitutional treatment only.

The prominent symptoms of the climacteric were as follows: Marked debility, 24; intense nervousness, 31; nervous prostration, 9; melancholia, 10; headache, 14; neuralgia, 6; hysteria, 7; irritable heart, 11; tachycardia, 8; insomnia, 19; indigestion, 32; constipation, 28; diarrhea, 3; leucorrhea, 38; rheumatism, 21; gout, 1; Bright's disease, 12; hemorrhage, 6; alcoholism, 2; corpulency, 2.

As a result of the study of these cases, the most striking feature was the relation of miscarriages to the sufferings and ill health at the time of the menopause. Of the nineteen women who had miscarriages, only one did not suffer in some way at the time of the menopause. Four suffered only slightly, and fourteen suffered extremely, not only during the menopause, but in the post-climacteric period as well. And the next most striking feature was that the prominent symptoms of the menopause are preeminently reflex or the functional diseases of the nervous system.

Tilt believes that single women suffer less than other women at the time of the menopause. He further writes: "As at puberty, from the ignorance in which it is still thought right to leave young women, so at the change of life, women often suffer from ignorance of what may occur, or from exaggerated notions of the perils which await them. It would be well if they were made to understand that if in tolerable health, provided that they will conform to judicious rules, they have only blessings to expect from the change of life. Most unfortunately, the individual not cognizant of the invisible changes going on in the economy does not adapt the mode of life to the new conditions of the organism, and the weakened and lessened amount of the digestive fluids is unable to master the large quantities of food. The absorbents refuse to take more than is needed to repair the tissues. The atrophying muscles of the digestive tube, unable to hurry on the mixed products of indigestion; fermentation; and micro-organisms inciting fermentations and elaborating toxic alkaloids, poison and disorder the functions of life. Man's outdoor life enables him to escape many of these evils.

"Woman's enervating mode of life, the continued introspection, coupled with the peculiar changes in the nutrition of the body at this time, render the nervous system peculiarly impressionable and liable to the manifold forms of diseases. 'The woman is told that she must be calm and patient, and in time the tomb-builder will alleviate all her sufferings.' This critical period may be dangerous to those who are always ailing, for habitiual sufferers at the menstrual periods, and for those affected with uterine diseases. If, on the first indication of the change of life, women who are in fair health carefully followed a regimen and pursued a line of life in harmony with the physiologic processes on which this change depends, disease would be prevented. But as the change concerns a natural function, it is left to nature; no additional precautions are taken, and advice is sought only when the mischief is done."

It is not wise to marry during this period. On the first appearance of the irregularities of the menopause the amount of food and stimulants to which women have been accustomed should be curtailed rather than augmented. The system requires supporting by medicine and regimen— as, baths, mental and moral hygiene, and occupation— rather than stimulating by spirits.

We have seen that, in accordance with the plethric theory, which prevailed until 1835, and with the nerve theory, which is based on the latest anatomic and physiologic researches, menstruation is a physiologic process to get rid of effete material, and is therefore an excretion.

At the end of perhaps thirty years, by a conservative process of nature, the child-bearing period ceases and the organism is readjusted to the end that the woman's vitality may all be conserved for her own individual life.

Each metamorphic or developmental period of life— dentition, puberty, and the menopause— throws a special strain on the nervous system, and the recent studies of the sympathetic nervous system at the time of the menopause show that very extensive anatomic changes occur at this time. That being the case, the woman must lead such a life as will insure her having on hand a large reserve force necessary to meet these heavy demands. Tilt's observations show that women who have experienced no suffering at puberty or, at the menstrual periods do not suffer at the menopause. It is therefore evident that the time to begin this preparation is in childhood.

That single women suffer less than married women would suggest that excessive coitus and the occurrence of abortions, frequent child-bearing, and lesions as the result of pregnancies, many of which lesions could have been prevented or cured by the timely aid of the physician, are the combined sources of much of the suffering at the time of the menopause.

That the most frequent and serious disturbances are those of the nervous system, and that from their mode of life and habits of introspection the rich suffer more from these ailments than the poor, must cause serious consideration of the physiologic necessity for a definite occupation for the daughters as well as for the sons of the rich.

The frequency with which Bright's disease is found at the time of the menopause is dependent not so much on the local physiologic changes which are taking place as on the time of life. Loomis says that it was not until life-insurance examinations became so common that the frequency with which kidney disease existed in persons who believed themselves well was even imagined. And as a result of his observations in these cases, and of a large number of autopsies conducted at the Bellevue, he stated that it was his belief that 90% of men and women over forty years of age suffer from some form of Bright's disease. That being the case, it would seem that after this period of life at least as much attention should be directed to the kidneys as to the teeth, and that a semi-annual examination of the urine should be made.

Although the menopause is a physiologic occurrence, yet, owing to the many pathologic changes which are liable to take place at this time, the woman should be as carefully watched during the menopause by the gynecologist as the pregnant woman now is by the obstetrician. If the same care were taken, in the majority of cases, the dangers attending the menopause would be avoided, and the woman would be prepared to enjoy a healthy and useful post-climacteric period of life.

CHAPTER XV.

HYGIENE OF THE MENOPAUSE.

Diet; Constipation; Stimulants; the Kidneys; the Skin; Turkish Baths; Massage; Exercise; Profuse Menstruation; Hemorrhage; Mental Therapeutics.

> "'Tis the breathing time of day."
>
> — *"Hamlet."*

Hygiene of the Menopause.— The changes which occur in all the organs of the body at the time of the menopause are retrograde, and therefore just the opposite of those which occur at the time of puberty. This fact should be borne in mind in the matter of alimentation. All that is now needed is to make the repair equal to the waste.

Diet.— Unless the woman is taking a great deal of active exercise, it is better to diminish the amount of meat eaten, and to increase the vegetable food and take more fluids. Unless the effect of the meat eaten is counterbalanced by active outdoor exercise, it produces an excess of waste matter, which accumulates and causes biliousness, and sometimes rheumatism and gout. A vegetable diet is less taxing to the excretory organs than an animal diet.

Indigestion is at this time of life apt to appear in the form of fermentation, which may assume the gastric or intestinal type. The chief causes of the formation of gases are the lessened peristaltic action of the intestines, the increased tendency to congestion of the liver and to obstinate constipation.

All dishes rich in sugar, as cake, candy, preserves, and jelly, should be indulged in with moderation; or where there is a tendency to fermentative indigestion, they should be wholly avoided.

All dishes known to be difficult of digestion, as hot breads, pastry, cheese, fried dishes, and rich salads, should be cut off the menu, since these readily overtax an already weakened digestive system.

If there is a hereditary tendency to rheumatism or gout, the disease is most apt to take on an active form at this time. In either case the manifestation of the disease indicates an excess of uric acid in the system, and a diet becomes a necessity. Pickles, all highly spiced articles of food, and vinegar must be omitted from the bill of fare. The vinegar may be replaced in salad-dressings by lemon juice. Tomatoes, rhubarb, strawberries and grapefruit are contraindicated; also all articles of food rich in sugar.

In chronic cases animal food cannot, as a rule, be excluded from the dietary, but must be limited in quantity. Fish, eggs, and fowl may be eaten, also a moderate amount of lean meat in the form of beef, lamb, and mutton. Milk may be indulged in freely. The diet should consist principally of easily digested fresh green vegetables. The amount of tea and coffee should be limited. All malt liquors, sweet wines, and champagne must be absolutely prohibited.

Constipation.— A daily free evacuation of the bowels is essential to good health. Where constipation exists, and the woman is full-blooded, with a tendency to a rush of blood to the head, saline laxatives are indicated. But if the woman is constipated and anemic, cascara sagrada is a better laxative; while cod-liver oil acts as a laxative and at the same time improves the quality of the blood.

Stimulants.— Women resort to alcoholic stimulants as an analgesic to relieve pain, whether physical or mental; as a narcotic to produce sleep; and as a spur to a failing appetite or bodily powers.

The majority of women patients say that they first used alcohol in the shape of whisky, brandy or gin to relieve pain at the time of the menstrual period. The pain that is caused at this time by a chilling of the body would be as effectually relieved by drinking a cup of hot tea; while if the pain is intense and constant, recurring every month, it is doubtless caused by some local inflammation, and the use of alcohol only veils the real trouble, and the woman loses valuable time by not consulting a physician at once.

As to the use of alcohol to blunt the nervous sensibility due to mental suffering, it is the testimony of the entire medical profession that this is the greatest cause of inebriety or drunkenness among women of all classes of society.

Sleeplessness generally arises from some well-defined physical cause— very frequently from inaction of the liver— and the proper remedial agents should be used to remove the cause.

While at first the use of alcoholic beverages increases the appetite, as the amount taken is increased, distaste for food is created, the system languishes under an insufficient food-supply, and the original aim of increasing the appetite is defeated.

As to taking stimulants to do more work than one could otherwise accomplish, it is by means of stimulants that woman can accomplish her physiological ruin more quickly than is possible in any other way. And the early symptoms of chronic alcoholism show themselves in the form of neuralgia, insomnia, palpitation of the heart, and muscular tremors.

The Kidneys.— On account of the prevalence of some form of Bright's disease after forty years of life, the kidneys should be carefully watched at this time. And in order to keep them in good condition they must be well flushed with water every day. Three pints of urine should be excreted daily, and three pints of water as such must be taken into the system daily. The urine should be examined by the physician every six months. In this way kidney disease is often discovered in its incipiency, which otherwise might run into a serious form of Bright's disease.

The Skin.— It must be remembered that the skin is one of the excretory organs of the body, and the pores should be kept well open by the various forms of baths.

The Turkish bath or some modification of it will often be found to be particularly useful. Massage with alcohol after the bath lessens the tendency to take cold. For a woman who is anemic or run down, it is well to follow the Turkish with the Roman bath, which is an inunction with almond oil or cocoa-butter. A much more thorough massage is given with the Roman bath than with the "alcohol rub." It is often necessary to modify the Turkish bath by omitting the steam-room and shortening the time spent in the hot dry air. In ordinary cases the time spent in the hot dry-room should be only that necessary for producing a free perspiration. This time varies in different individuals from ten to twenty minutes. No woman should go to a Turkish bath without first consulting her physician, since if the woman has a weak heart, the bath may be the source of positive danger. Comparatively few women are strong enough to take the cold plunge.

Massage. — Massage, well given by a skilful masseuse twice a week, will greatly tone up the nervous and circulatory systems. Women who are very stout and who have sluggish livers with obstinate constipation will find massage particularly beneficial.

Exercise. — Daily exercise in the open air is absolutely essential to every woman's good health. The minimum amount of outdoor exercise compatible with health is an hour's walk, at the rate of three miles an hour. If the woman has never taken any exercise, she must begin with a very short walk and stop on the first sign of fatigue. Gradually increase the distance and the speed until the three miles is reached.

Profuse Menstruation. — If the menstrual flow is unusually profuse or lasts beyond the regular time, the woman should stay quietly in bed until the flow ceases. All exercise increases the flow.

The flow now becomes less in quantity, and the periods more infrequent than formerly. *Hemorrhage* must always be regarded as a danger-signal the significance of which can scarcely be overestimated. To immediately consult a specialist on the appearance of any irregularities of the flow would, in the opinion of the most eminent gynecologists of the day, be the means of saving thousands of women's lives every year.

Mental Therapeutics. — It is particularly necessary at this time of life that the mind should be pleasantly occupied. Her children have passed the age when they need her constant supervision, and the mother must take some relaxation from her home cares, in the form of social diversions, amusements, outdoor life, and change of scene. Any mental occupation that will take the woman out of herself is the best possible safeguard against a state of introspection which conjures up a host of evil fantasies, and which is the first step in the downward road to a fixed and permanent melancholia.

> "Hang sorrow, care will kill a cat;
> And therefore let 's be merry."

CHAPTER XVI.

HINTS FOR HOME TREATMENT

Indigestion; Constipation; Diarrhea; Enemas; Vaginal Douche; Baths; Headache; Fainting; Hemorrhage.

> "Woman is woman's natural ally."
>
> — EURIPIDES.

Indigestion. — The chief causes of indigestion are: eating rapidly, eating at irregular hours, eating indigestible foods, constipation, and lack of exercise. No one who values her good health will allow herself to be hurried through a meal, nor will she allow the perplexities of life to be thrust upon her at the table for solution. The first requisite for the digestion of foods is that they should be well masticated, so that the digestive fluids may act on the finely divided particles to the greatest possible advantage. And while digestion is going on all mental labor should be held in abeyance, in order to avoid drawing the blood away from the stomach to the brain. Furthermore, it is a well-known fact that digestion is best performed when the meals are served at regular hours.

Constipation leads to the formation of gases in the intestines, to fermentation, and to the absorption of toxic materials by the blood.

Through lack of exercise, the appetite fails, the liver becomes torpid, and the muscular and nervous systems lose their tone.

The exercise which the housekeeper gets in going around her house is not sufficient. Daily exercise in the open air is essential to health; as this is to supplement the indoor exercise, the amount taken will vary in proportion to the former. For teachers or those who have a sedentary occupation an hour's active exercise in the open air— a three-mile walk— should be supplemented by active gymnastic exercise.

For people in good health, a mixed diet— that is to say, a diet consisting of meat, vegetables, and fruit— is the best. If the individual is not well, then the diet must be adapted to meet the needs of that particular case.

Hot breads, all articles of food fried in fats, salads, and pastry are difficult to digest. Tea is very constipating, and when taken in excessive quantities renders the individual nervous. An excess of coffee leads to congestion of the liver.

Where indigestion exists, the simplest and most sensible remedies are to regulate the diet, and avoid eating between meals. By drinking a glass of water as hot as it can be sipped one hour before each meal, the mucus is washed out of the stomach, the stomach is empty on coming to the table, and in the best possible condition for the gastric juice to act on the food-stuffs.

Constipation.— Constipation is the rule with the average American woman; the causes are their corsets, the tight bands of their clothing, lack of exercise, and the fact that they drink too little water and too much tea. The most rational means to overcome it is to drink more water; at least three pints a day should be taken, in addition to soups, tea and coffee, and so forth; the water must be taken into the system as such. Then attention must be given to the diet; plenty of fruit should be eaten, vegetables, and coarse bread.

Regularity in this, as in all other habits of life, is most essential, and the individual should go to the toilet at the same hour every day, even if there is no inclination to have a bowel movement, and thus the habit will be established; the most convenient time is directly after breakfast.

Medical Treatment. — But if all these means have failed, medicines must be resorted to. Cold water is a better laxative than hot; to a glassful of cold water add from one teaspoonful to one tablespoonful of the effervescing granules of the phosphate of soda, and take this the first thing on rising in the morning. This preparation of soda is particularly useful because it acts slightly on the liver. Other laxatives are: a seidlitz powder dissolved in a glass of cold water on rising; a wineglass or more of Hunyadi Janos, also taken on rising. Any of these may be taken with safety by pregnant women. For children the simplest laxative is one teaspoonful of Husband's milk of magnesia, to be taken in one glass of water on rising.

Enemas.— Perhaps one of the most common methods used by the laity for the relief of constipation is the rectal injection, or enema. Enemas habitually given to unload the bowels are productive of much harm by overdistending the rectum, so that in time the rectum fails to react to the normal stimulus— namely, the presence of the feces— as it otherwise would. But by some means or other the bowels must be well moved once every twenty-four hours. And it is much better to use an enema than to go to bed without a bowel movement. If the woman is going around, so that she can give the enema to herself, the most effective way to take it is in the knee-chest position or an approximation to this. Either a fountain or bulb syringe may be used for this purpose; a quart of water at a temperature of 110° F. should be prepared by making it into a suds with castile soap, or one tablespoonful of glycerin may be added to one pint of water. The nozle to be used is the smallest one that comes with the syringe, the so-called infant's nozle; this is quite large enough, and its insertion is not nearly so painful as the larger ones; the nozle must be well greased with vaselin. When everything is ready, the patient gets down on her knees with the shoulders near the floor, having first loosened all of her bands and taken off her corsets; the nozle is introduced as far as it will go into the rectum, and if a bulb syringe is used the water must be very gradually squeezed into the rectum, otherwise it will not retain so much; or if the fountain syringe is used, it must not be hung too high. So soon as the patient feels that she has taken all that she can retain, she should lie down on the left side, and retain the water as long as possible, as it is thus rendered more effective. An enema so taken will be very much more effective than one taken in the ordinary manner of sitting on the toilet. In the method just described more water can be used and it will be longer retained; it can be felt to go up along the course of the large bowel, and it will often be found very effective when the ordinary enema fails. This enema will often be found to be a very valuable aid in curing an obstinate chronic diarrhea, which is kept up by particles of feces remaining in the folds of the large intestine. If the patient is confined to bed, she should lie on the left side, with a heavy towel folded under her to prevent the bed from becoming wet; when the nurse withdraws the nozle she should make pressure on the anus with the towel, to help the patient to retain the water as long as possible. But should the patient have gone so long without a bowel movement that all these means fail, it will be necessary to precede the water enema with one of oil; or still more effective is the following combination: take one teaspoonful of the spirits of turpentine, the yolk of one egg, and two tablespoonfuls of olive oil, and beat well together, and add to these one pint of water at a temperature of 110° F. Constipation, however, of so obstinate a character as this demands a physician's attention.

Diarrhea. — A diarrhea may be acute or chronic; the treatment is essentially different. For an acute attack accompanied by frequent stools and severe abdominal pain the first thing to do is to go to bed. If there is nausea, drink a glass of water as hot as can be taken, at once; for the diet, a glass of scalded milk, not boiled but just allowed to come to the boiling-point, every two hours; and nothing else should be taken until the diarrhea is well in check. If the pain is severe, a spice plaster over the abdomen will be found to be very comforting. It is made as follows: take of powdered allspice, cinnamon, cloves, and ginger each two tablespoonfuls, and two teaspoonfuls of cayenne pepper; mix well together in a bowl; then quilt in a piece of flannel large enough to cover the abdomen; when ready for use, dip in hot whisky and apply as hot as the patient can bear; cover over with a large napkin, as the plaster produces a deep stain which does not wash out; keep on as long as necessary. If the rest in bed and the milk diet kept up for twenty-four hours do not suffice to cure the diarrhea, it is not wise to take any risks, but send for your doctor at once. Or if there should be any blood in the stools, do not wait for anything, but send for the doctor without delay.

For a chronic diarrhea an enema given in the knee-chest position, as already described, will often be found a most efficient remedy. In diarrheas the use of fruits and vegetables should be avoided; the best diet after the milk is bread well toasted through, toast-water, soft-boiled eggs, beefsteak, oyster stew, and clam broth.

Vaginal Douche.— To be of service except for mere cleansing purposes the douche must be taken in the horizontal position, either on a couch or, if it is not cold, on the floor. Of course, this position necessitates the use of a douche-pan. The douche-pan is best of agate-ware, oblong in shape, and with a broad strip which comes under the nates. On lying down to take the douche the nates must come down well over the pan and the clothing must be pushed well up to prevent the water from seeping up the back. To make the woman more comfortable there should be a pillow under the head, and she must have a shawl or some light woolen material to throw over her while taking the douche to prevent chilling; thus doing more harm than good.

There are two forms of syringes on the market: the bag or fountain syringe, which is hung up sufficiently high— about three feet above the patient— to cause the water to flow; and the bulb syringe, in which the bulb has to be constantly squeezed by the hand, which is tiresome to many women, but this is a much more convenient form to have in traveling. During pregnancy the fountain syringe only should be used, and it should be hung as low as will enable the water to flow. For a woman who has never taken douches it is well to begin with a temperature of 110° F., gradually increasing the temperature to 118° or 120°; this is as high as the woman should attempt to go, for a higher temperature would burn her, leaving the vulva so sensitive that she would only be able to take cool douches for a long time after this; a bath thermometer should be used in all cases to test the temperature, so that the woman knows exactly what she is doing.

In cases of inflammation of the uterus or its adnexa four quarts of water should be used, and the douche should be taken in the horizontal position. The water thus acts as a hot poultice about the uterus, and the woman will find on rising that some water flows out from the vagina. Ordinarily plain hot water is all that is necessary to use, but where the discharge is acrid and scalding, the plain hot-water douche should be followed by a warm douche containing one teaspoonful of borax to a pint of water. The best time for taking a douche is at night just before retiring; there is also less danger of taking cold when the douche is taken at this time.

The scalding sensations at the vulva may be due to the acidity of the urine, in which case it will be increased just after urination; or it may be due to an acrid discharge from the vagina. A little observation on the part of the patient will enable her to distinguish which is the real cause. If there is any trouble with the urine, it should be carefully examined at once, as some congestion or inflammation of the kidneys is not infrequently present, which if attended to might be cured, and which if allowed to run on unattended to, may develop into a serious form of Bright's disease.

The genitals should be washed with soap and water night and morning. Women who do not suffer from leuchorrhea need not take a vaginal douche more than once a week; after the menstrual flow the vaginal injection is advised to remove the detritus of the flow.

Baths.— The most ordinary forms of baths used may be classified under sponge-, shower-, sitz-, and tub-baths. The sponge-bath as ordinarily taken is of service for cleansing purposes, and if the water be cold it tones up the system to some extent, and is so a preventive against taking cold. The effect of this bath will be found to be vastly more beneficial if salt is added to the bath in the proportion of a pint of salt to a gallon of water; either sea-salt may be used or the ordinary coarse salt. It is most advantageously taken sitting in a bath or hat-tub, so that the entire surface of the body will be wet at the same time, and the water can be allowed to run down the back and over the chest. It is well to begin these baths at a temperature of 80° F. and to gradually decrease this until the bath is taken at 70°, which is about the temperature of running water, and the bath should be kept up at this. For most people the best time to take the bath is just before retiring; this bath is not only very strengthening, but also is excellent in cases of insomnia and nervousness.

Shower-baths.— These may be taken after a hot bath, or taken alone after violent muscular exercise. The body should be quickly scrubbed off and the shower should be warm at the beginning and gradually allowed to become cold, stooping over so as to get the full force of the shower on the spine and over the region of the stomach and heart. They will be found to be most refreshing after great muscular fatigue, and, when taken after the hot tub-bath, greatly lessen the susceptibility of the individual to taking cold.

Sitz-baths. – These are given for their local effect in cases of inflammation; whether this inflammation be of the kidneys, bladder, or of the uterus and its adnexa. A sitz-tub is necessary to properly take this form of bath. The water should be used as hot as is comfortable to the patient, from 105° to 110° F., hot water being added as the first cools off; a pint of salt should be added to the gallon of water, and the patient should remain in this from five to eight minutes. A blanket should be wrapped about the patient so that she will be thrown into a perspiration; it is almost needless to say that the only time for taking this bath is just before retiring, and that this bath does make the woman more susceptible to taking cold, so that it is necessary to wear an abdominal woolen bandage day and night.

Tub-baths. – The tub-bath ought not, as a rule, be taken more than twice a week, unless the cold plunge is used, which may be taken every day. If the tub-bath is taken hot, the woman should remain in it not much longer than is necessary to scrub off with a flesh-brush; this bath should be followed either with a cold shower-bath, or the water in the tub be gradually allowed to cool off until it is down to 70° F.

Headaches. – Headaches, aside from those of acute illness, may be roughly divided into three classes: first, those which are due to indigestion; second, neuralgic headaches; and, third, those due to pelvic inflammations. The headaches due to indigestion are usually located over the eyes and all over the forehead; they are more or less constant and are accompanied by other symptoms of indigestion, and very often by constipation. The feces are allowed to remain in the bowels overlong, the toxic matters are taken up by the blood, and headaches and vertigo result.

Neuralgic headaches are of an entirely different character; the pains are here of a lancinating character, and are not confined to any one region of the head. As a rule, they are accompanied by neuralgic pains in other parts of the body. Neuralgia generally means a rundown state of the system from overwork, worry, or malaria, and tonics and cod-deliver oil are indicated.

A constant dull pain on the top of the head or in the back of the neck generally indicates some uterine inflammation, and can only be cured by removing the cause. In any case it is very evident that taking the various "headache powders" with which the market is flooded will never cure the woman of her headaches; and many of these powders are very dangerous, especially where the heart is weak, as most of them are heart-depressants.

Fainting.— Fainting may be due to a weak heart, to heart disease, or to sudden shock, as on receiving a bad piece of news; during pregnancy the close air of a room may cause a woman to faint. The first thing to be done is to lay the woman down on the floor or bed with nothing under her head; loosen all her clothes about the neck and waist, and throw the windows open so that she will get plenty of fresh air. If she is able to drink, give her one teaspoonful of aromatic spirits of ammonia in four tablespoonfuls of cold water. If the feet are cold, place hot-water bottles to them to improve the circulation. And if at the end of fifteen minutes she does not show signs of decided improvement, give her two tablespoonfuls of whisky in an equal quantity of hot water. In the meantime the physician will have been summoned. These attacks of fainting often occur in a crowded ball-room, and are due to tight lacing and the poor ventilation of the room.

Hemorrhage.— A profuse hemorrhage is the most alarming as well as the most dangerous thing which can befall a woman, and the very nearest doctor should be summoned until the family physician can be gotten there. The woman should be made to lie down wherever she may happen to be, her clothes loosened, the windows thrown open, so that she will not only have plenty of fresh air, but that the air shall be cool. If the blood is coming from the mouth, give her pieces of ice to hold in it; if she coughs up the blood, it would be well to put a bag of ice-cold water or cloths wrung out of ice-water on the chest. If the woman is suffering from a uterine hemorrhage, have her take at once a hot vaginal douche, from 118° to 120° F., and have the foot of the bed raised. The head should always be kept low.

Women hold their health in their own hands to a far greater extent than they have ever dreamed of; and if the majority of women suffer, it is very often their own fault, either because they have disregarded nearly every law of health, or have allowed trivial ailments to go on until they were almost incurable.

> "The broad mountain-top, with its sunlight and free air, is possible to all of us, if we choose to struggle on and reach it."
>
> — Phillips Brooks.

GLOSSARY.

Abortion. The expulsion of the fetus before the end of the third lunar month.

Afferent Nerves. Those nerves which convey the impressions to the nerve-centers.

After-pains. The pains which follow labor and which are caused by the contractions of the uterus.

Amenorrhea. Absence of the menstrual flow.

Anemia. The so-called thinness of the blood, due to a deficiency of red blood-corpuscles.

Antisepsis. The use of chemical substances which have the power of destroying germs.

Anus. The external circular outlet of the rectum or distal part of the large intestine.

Appendages, Uterine. The Fallopian tubes, the ligaments of the uterus, and the ovaries.

Atrophy. A progressive diminution in the bulk of an organ or tissue.

Automatic. Involuntary, mechanical.

Bulbi Vestibuli. A plexus of veins on each side of the vestibule.

Capillaries. The terminal and very finest branches of the blood-vessels.

Catamenial Flow. See *Menstruation*.

Cellular Tissue. A loose, transparent tissue which surrounds the muscles and organs of the body.

Cerebrum. The upper and larger portion of the brain.

Chlorosis. Anemia of young women about the time of puberty.

Climacteric. See *Menopause*.

Clitoris. A small, elongated, erectile organ situated at the upper part of the vulva.

Cohabitation. See *Coitus*.

Coition. See *Coitus*.

Coitus. Syn., coition, copulation, cohabitation, sexual congress, sexual intercourse. The carnal union of the sexes.

Colostrum. A thin albuminous fluid which appears in the breasts at the fourth month of pregnancy.

Conception, or impregnation, is the union of the germ and sperm cell which results in a new being.
Confinement. Childbed, the expulsion of the child from the womb.
Congestion. The abnormal accumulation of blood in a part.
Constipation. Costiveness; a state in which there is not a free daily evacuation of the bowels, or where the evacuations are hard or expelled with difficulty.
Continence. Abstinence from or moderation in sexual indulgence.
Copulation. See *Coitus.*
Cord, Umbilical. The cord which connects the fetus with the mother. Through the blood-vessels contained in this cord the child receives nourishment.
Corpuscle. A very small particle.

Decidua. A membranous sac formed in the uterus during gestation, and thrown off after parturition.
Defecation. The act by which the contents of the bowel are expelled from the body.
Dehiscence. The splitting open of an organ.
Dentition. The cutting of the teeth.
Dysmenorrhea. Painful and difficult menstruation.
Dystocia. A difficult labor.

Embryo. The name applied to the very earliest stages of the child in utero; that is, up to about the time of quickening.
Endometrium. The lining membrane of the uterus.
Epithelium. A layer of minute cells which forms the covering of many membranes.
Erection. The state of a part which, having been soft, becomes rigid and elevated by the accumulation of blood within its tissues.

Fallopian Tubes. Two very small tubes extending from the upper angles of the uterus to the ovaries and serving to convey the ova from the ovaries to the uterus.
Feces. Stools; the normal discharge from the bowels.
Fetus. The child in utero from the time of quickening to that of birth.
Fomentations. The application of cloths which have previously been dipped in hot water.

Function. An action of an organ which could be performed only by that organ, and which is necessary to the well-being of the individual.

Generative Organs. Syn., genital, reproductive, sexual; those organs in the male and female by means of which a new being is created.
Genital. See *Generative*.
Gestation. See *pregnancy*.
Gonorrhea. A highly contagious venereal disease, characterized by an inflammatory discharge of mucus from the urethra and prepuce in the male, and from the urethra and the vagina in the female.
Graafian Follicles. Minute ovarian vesicles which contain the ova.

Hemorrhoids. Piles or tumors at or within the anus, and consisting of enlarged veins.
Hymen. The semilunar fold situated at the outer orifice of the vagina in the virgin.
Hypertrophy. The increased activity of a part which leads to an increase in its bulk.
Hypochondriasis. Morbid feelings concerning the health and simulating disease.

Impregnation. See *Conception*.
Infectious. See *Contagious*.

Katabolic Nerves are those nerves which stimulate the breaking down of tissue.

Labia Majora. Two thick folds of skin which extend backward from the mons veneris.
Labia Minora. Nymphae; two very delicate folds of skin which are inside of and protected by the labia majora.
Labor. See *Parturition*.
Lactation. The secretion of milk; nursing, suckling the child.
Lactiferous Ducts. The milk ducts.
Leucorrhea. Whites; a whitish or yellowish discharge from the vagina.
Lochia. A discharge which follows labor and which lasts for about two weeks.

Lying-in. The period which follows childbed.
Lymphatics. The vessels in which the lymph is carried.

Mammae. The mammary glands; the breasts.
Marital Relations. See *Coitus*.
Massage. A systematic kneading of the muscles.
Meatus Urinarius. The external orifice of the urethra.
Meconium. The first discharge from the infant's bowel after birth, and which had collected in the intestines during the pregnancy.
Medulla. The base of the brain at its junction with the spinal cord.
Menopause. Climacteric, change of life, the time of the natural cessation of the monthly sickness.
Menorrhagia. An excessive menstrual flow.
Menstruation. Menstrual period, menstrual flow, menses, monthly sickness, the monthly discharge of blood from the uterus, which, with certain exceptions, recurs monthly from about the age of thirteen to forty-six years.
Metabolism. Transformation changes.
Metamorphoses. Changes of shape or structure.
Metrorrhagia. A flow of blood between the menstrual periods.
Micturition. The act of passing water.
Miscarriage. The expulsion of the fetus between the twelfth and twenty-eighth weeks.
Molecular. Belonging to the molecules, or the minutest portion of anything.
Mons Veneris. The uppermost part of the vulva, which is a fatty cushion covered with hair.

Nerve-center. A nerve station from which orders are transmitted and where orders are received.
Nubile. Puberty, that period of life in which young people of both sexes are capable of procreating children.
Nymphae. See *Labia minora*.

Ovaries. Two small ovoid bodies, one on each side of the uterus, in which the ova are formed.
Oviduct. See *Fallopian tobe*.
Ovulation. The formation of the ova in the ovary, and the discharge of the same.

Ovule. See *Ovum*.
Ovum. Germ cell, a small, round vesicle situated in the ovaries, and which, when fecundated, constitutes the rudiments of the embryo.

Parturition. Labor, delivery, child-birth, the expulsion of the child from the womb.
Pathologic. Relating to the diseased condition of tie body.
Pelvis. The bony cavity situated at the lower end of the spinal column and supported by the thighs.
Periodicity. The recurrence of physiologic phenomena at regular intervals.
Periphery. The circumference of an organ.
Peristaltic Action. An alternate contraction, making small, and enlargement of the bowel; it is by this means that foods, etc., are forced along its passage.
Peritoneum. A serous membrane which lines the abdominal cavity, and wholly or in part envelopes the organs contained in it; it also partly covers the organs contained in the pelvic cavity.
Phenomena. Remarkable appearances.
Physical. Pertaining to the body.
Placenta. After-birth, a soft, spongy, vascular body adherent to the uterus, and which is connected with the embryo through the umbilical cord.
Plethora. A condition marked by a superabundance of blood.
Postpartum Hemorrhage. Hemorrhage following labor.
Pregnant. Enceinte, gravid; the state of a woman who is with child.
Premature Labor. The expulsion of the fetus between the end of the twenty-eighth week and the time that labor ought to have occurred.
Propagation. The spreading or extension of a thing.
Pruritus Vulva. An intense itching of the privates, or vulva.
Psychic. Pertaining or belonging to the mind.
Puberty. Sexual maturity; nubility; that period of life in which young people of both sexes are capable of procreating children.
Pubes or Pubis. The lowest and middle part of the pelvis in its anterior surface.
Puerperium. The lying-in after child-birth.

Quickening. The sensation experienced by the mother as the result of active fetal movements in the womb.

Rectum. The lower extremity of the large intestine.
Reflex. The reflection of an impulse from a nerve-center which has been received from elsewhere by that center.
Reproduction. See *Generative*.
Respiration. Breathing.
Rugs. Wrinkles.
Rut. The copulation of animals.

Septicemia, Puerperal. Childbed fever.
Sexual. That which relates to sex. See *Generative*.
Smegma. A cheesy substance which may collect about the vulva.
Spermatozoa. The essential male fertilizing elements.
Sympathetic Nervous System. Presides over involuntary acts; as digestion, breathing, etc.
Syphilis. A venereal disease which is highly contagious by coition, contact with the lips, etc.

Tachycardia. Distress in the region of the heart, with palpitation and shortness of breath.

Umbilicus. Navel.
Urea. The most important of the solid constituents of the urine.
Ureters. The ducts leading from the kidneys to the bladder.
Urethra. The excretory duct from the bladder for the escape of the urine.
Urination. The act of passing water.
Uterosacral Ligaments. Ligaments which pass from the uterus to the sacrum, and assist in holding the uterus in position.
Uterus. Womb; the hollow, pear-shaped pelvic organ which is destined to retain the child from the moment of its conception until the time of its expulsion at birth.
Utricular Glands. Glands of the uterus.

Vagina. The canal which connects the female internal and external organs of generation.
Vascular. Pertaining to the blood-vessels.
Vasomotor Nervous System. Comprises the brain, spinal cord, and the nerves given off from the cord: this system presides over volun-

tary acts, that is, those acts which are under the control of the will.
Vestibule. A smooth cavity that exists in the female between the perineum and the nymphae.
Viscera. The contents of the large cavities of the body.
Vulva. The external genitals, private parts, the female external organs of generation.
Vulvitis. Inflammation of the vulva.

www.ingramcontent.com/pod-product-compliance
Lightning Source LLC
Chambersburg PA
CBHW031418210526
45464CB00005B/1945